The Divine Farmer's Renga

A Materia Medica of Chinese Herbal Medicine and Haiku

Alexander Lucksmith

With illustrations by Camino F.

The information herein is for entertainment purposes only and should
not be taken as medical advice. Consult a licensed health care
practitioner if seeking diagnosis or treatment. As Doc said "the doctor
who treats himself is twice the fool".

Printed in the United States of America

First Printing, May 2015
Pigeonpine Press
Pigeonpine.com

To my friends on the other side:

Doc the Acupuncturist
Baisao and Steve, the Tea Sellers
Grandma the Librarian

Notes about this edition

You know those carved roadside sculptures of bears? The ones made out of old logs carved with a chainsaw. Their usually sold in the same places where you can buy Styrofoam tubs of nightcrawlers and beef jerky in tobacco chew canisters. Standing in a loose group underneath the price of diesel and phone cards, as if they were about to have a reunion photo taken. Some grinning with buck teeth, holding a salmon trophy aloft, some majestic and pastoral, and some so roughly cut that only imagination and sentimentality keep them from becoming kindling. That is what this book is; a family of pinewood ursa beaming with hope and pride by the highway onramp. Maybe in the future I'll have a lacquer of proper grammar and a gallery that doesn't also sell TruckNuts and nachos. But until then, you can find me covered in woodchips, smelling like labor, trying to carve my goofy smile into a hunk of wood.

If you know me personally, think of this book as my proxy. I might not be there in person to make you tea and tinctures, but you will always have me in stories. Hopefully I'll end up in your glovebox or carry-on bag as a passenger on your next journey. If you don't know me, by the time you finish this book I am sure we will be fast friends and I'm looking forward to the adventures we will surely have.

With love across the oceans,
Alex "Lucksmith" Pieroni

Introduction

My very first book on herbs and their uses is still one of my favorites. Gregory Tilford's Edible and Medicinal Plants of the West. It was not purchased for me and I'm not sure where it came from. In my mind it is one of those household goods that has no origin and is never replace, like an heirless heirloom. Whatever its origins, it came with me every weekend when we would head into the foothills outside of Denver. Fishing only yielded fish, and rock-hounding only yielded rocks, but plants could do anything. There were bluebells that tasted like oysters, groundcover with a crunch like a cucumber, and Shooting Stars with a tasty root, yet so small they did not "justify the death of these beautiful plants. I still have the same copy I've had since I was a kid. Every rip and fold only adding to how precious it is. Between the last page and the back cover is a stained imprint of what I swear still smells like yarrow.

I only trusted my amateur harvesting skills so much. When a book warns you that angelica root and water hemlock look nearly identical, you learn to avoid anything with a while umbrella of flowers. Luckily Denver, being in close proximity to the patchouli scented streets of Boulder, had enough natural grocers to supply me with all the herbs I needed. One particular grocer, now part of a much larger chain, had so many bins and tubs of plant parts that I had to find a new compendium to go with my travel-worn Tilford. I tried on a few different books, but like a good pair of shoes, you know the right thing when you see it. For me, it was a $3 copy of John Lust's "The Herb Book". Hundreds of herbs, dozens of formulas, recipes, dyes, lifestyle tips. This book brought herbalism from a weekend pastime to an aspirational lifestyle. At 15, with poor grades and a long-term plan of "graduate and move to a monastery in Japan", this became a lifeline to a less robe-wearing future.

To be honest, it is a future I am still reaching for. After high school I followed a watercourse of change, and not often as a willing participant. Half way through college, I was getting antsy to get my hands back into bins of herbs. This time, I wanted to be on the side of the register that did not have me depositing my paycheck in exchange for plants. A too brief apprenticeship with the first registered Acupuncturist in Colorado opened a door for me that I will never forget. A door to a 600 square foot dispensary at the front of a Chinese medicine college in a bad part of town that I look back on as paradise. While I wasn't a student, I got to learn about the structures and mechanism that move the cosmic machines of Oriental medicine. I had walls of herbs and things we called herbs but were really bugs, rocks, and pieces of people all at my tasting disposal. I also had a library of professors from Yellow Emperors to Divine Farmers who all taught me so much. I did have two teachers in particular that I took classes with nearly every day. One was Chinese Natural Cures by Henry Lu and the other the Materia Medica by Dan Bensky. Two teachers I have never met in person with two different learning styles, both of which contributed greatly to this book and to my overall satisfaction with life.

Maybe hand in hand with my love for herbs and Chinese medicine is my love for haiku and renga. Like my herbal field guide, I am not sure where my passion for haiku came from. I suspect a 2nd grade poetry assignments and a gold star sticker may have something to do with it. Whatever the origin, I loved the puzzle of trying to condense thunderstorms into droplets that make the reader exclaim "it's raining!" Along with Kerouac's "Dharma Bums", Faubion Bower's haiku anthology is the only other book I take with me while traveling. Scrawled on its yellowing margins are dozens of haiku written from airplanes over Kyoto, in rest stops along I-25, and corporate hotel rooms in downtown Atlanta.

At the top of each entry in this book is the Pinyin name of the herb, aligned to the page edge for easy reference. Following that are the common English names, the Japanese Kampo name, and the Latin name. The next section, marked in italics, are the qualities and organ channels associated with the herb. Below that are a jumble of words that may or may not have anything to do with anything, but are generally arranged in what I intend to be a pleasing pattern. I've named this truncated renga a "san-ku". If you say it fast enough, "san-ku" sounds like "thank you" with a bit of an accent, which is exactly the feeling I want to express to these herbs, and to you dear reader. Wherever you find this book, I hope it inspires you find the same adventures, aspirations, and education that made its creation possible.

Index of Subjects

Herbs That Regulate the Qi

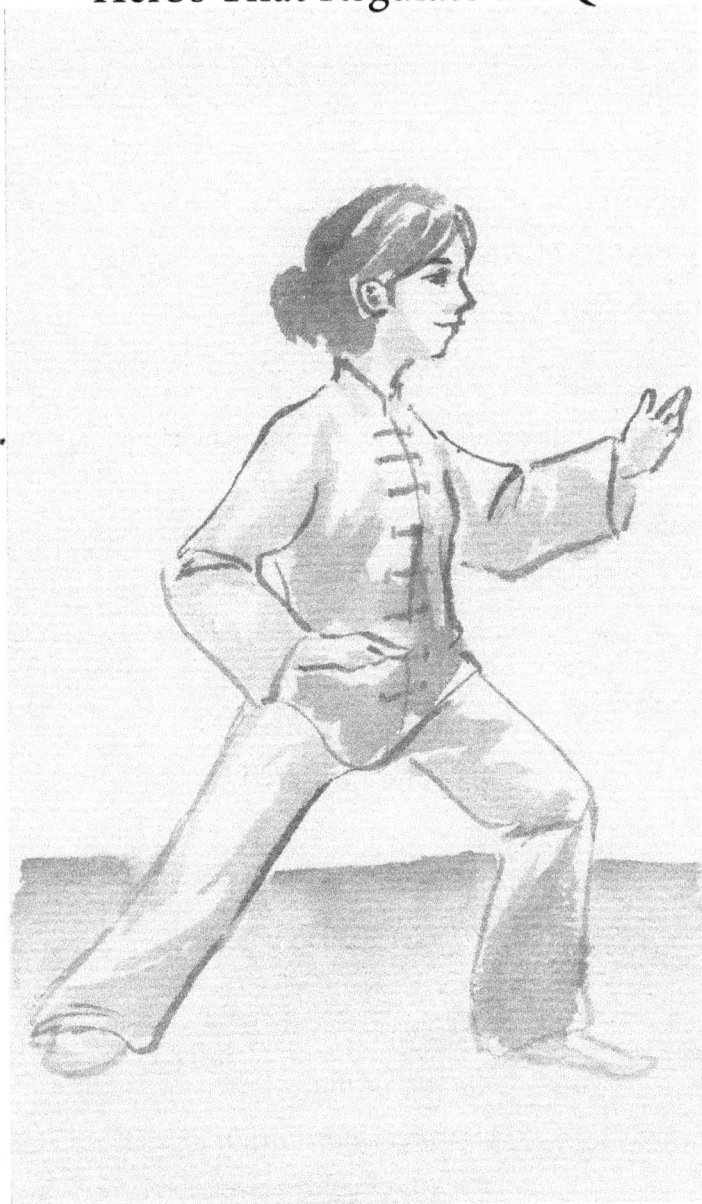

Chen Pi

Aged Tangerine peel
陳皮 (Chinpi)
Pericarpium Citri Reticulatae

Bitter, Spicy, Warm, Aromatic
LU, SP, ST

~ Regulates and descends Qi, improves transportive function in the middle Jiao, and relieves the diaphragm
~ Dries dampness and transforms phlegm
~ Prevents stagnation from tonic herbs

At the library
I see myself a bookworm
eating all I smell

A bookshelf of vintages
words ageing to perfection

Ink, paper, and glue
bound intoxication
gourmet information

Chen Xiang

Eaglewood, Aloeswood, Aquilaria
沈香 (Jinko)
Lignum Aquilariae Resinatum

Bitter, Spicy, Warm, Aromatic
KI, SP, ST

~ Promotes the movement of Qi and alleviates pain
~ Directs rebellious Qi downward, removes cold, warms the middle
  Jiao, and stops vomiting
~ Helps the kidneys grasp Qi and increases kidney warmth

In summer, hidden
in the winter, revealed
the eagles nest

It makes its home where it will
and no one dares disturb it

Talons and freedom
It is the perfect symbol
of our native land

Chuan Lian Zi

Sichuan Pagoda Tree, Sichuan Chinaberry, Melia
Fructus Toosendan

Bitter, Cold, Slightly Toxic
BL, LIV, SI, ST

~ Promotes the movement of Qi, dredges liver QI, guides out heat, and stops pain
~ Clears heat, dries dampness, regulates qi, alleviates pain due to damp-heat stagnant qi
~ Kills parasites and fungus and stops pain

---

1 p.m., wedding
at 3 p.m., funeral
6p.m., church

Shepard should be a title
like minister or servant

My old reverend;
a container for talents
Swiss-army person

Da Fu Pi

Betel husk

大腹皮 (Daifukuhi)

Pericarpium Arecae

Spicy, Slightly Warm
LI, SI, SP, ST

~ Promotes the downward movement of Qi and relaxes the middle Jiao
~ Expels damp, promotes urination and reduces edema

High schooler's party
I'm acting conspicuous
sipping from my flask

No one else needs to know
that I filled it with water

I wonder who else
is smoking oregano
and popping Red-Hots

Fo Shou

Finger Citron, Buddha's Hand Fruit
Fructus Citri Sarcodactylis

Bitter, Spicy, Warm
LI, LU, ST, SP

~ Regulates and soothes liver Qi
~ Harmonizes the stomach, strengthens the spleen, and dries dampness
~ Regulates lung QI and transforms phlegm

A hand that reaches
tree to the farmer
a hand that reaches

So much love he has for us
stretching forward from the green

I'm hesitating...
To chop the fingers from god
to garnish my tea...

Li Zhi He

Lychee nut
Semen Litchi

Sweet, Warm
LIV, ST

~ Regulates the Qi and stops pain
~ Disperses cold and stagnation, especially in the liver

With a single mind
he prepares the herb I seek
Hurls it from the tree

I wish I could understand
all the words you are saying

closed for winter
your wood-paneled office
is littered with shells

Mei Gui Hua

Asian Rosebud
Flos Rosae Rugosae

Sweet, Slightly Bitter, Warm
LIV, SP

~ Promotes the movement of Qi and relieves stagnation
~ Promotes the movement of Qi, harmonizes the blood, clears stasis, and regulates menstruation
~ Soothes the liver, eases pain, and dries diarrhea

In 29 years
I've never played so long
until I met you

I spilled my tea
when you told me I had a godson

We're hunting ghosts
with flashlights and stickers
endless poltergeists

16

Mu Xiang

Saussurea, Costus Root

木香 (Mokko)

Radix Aucklandiae

Bitter, Spicy, Warm
GB, LI, SP, ST

~ Promotes the movement of Qi and alleviates pain
~ Regulates stagnated Qi in the intestines
~ Clears damp heat and harmonizes liver and spleen
~ Strengthens the spleen and prevents stagnation

Bacon turn to wood
a container of slices
the apothecary wall

Every time I portion you
I think myself a butcher

Hunger quenched
with a tea made of breakfasts
Medicine as food

Qing Pi

Blue Citrus, Unripe Tangerine peel
Pericarpium Citri Reticulate Viride

Bitter, Spicy, Warm
GB, LIV, ST

~ Spreads liver Qi and breaks up stagnation
~ Reduces food stagnation and accumulations
~ Dries dampness and transforms phlegm

Abrasive flavor
Wincing from my harsh treatment
from a tiny dry medic

Resetting dislocation
is a violent affair

Soft words and aspirin
are of almost no comfort
when I'm unconscious

Shi Di

Kaki, Persimmon calyx
Calyx Kaki

Bitter, Astringent, Neutral
LU, ST

~   Descends stomach Qi downward

My heart in my throat
I see an Edo geisha
and my hiccups stop

Her white face a reflection
of my past and future lives

Who does she become
layers of silk on the floor,
Netflix on TV

Tan Xiang

Sandalwood, Chandana
Santanlum album

Spicy, Warm, Aromatic
LU, SP, ST

~ Promotes Qi movement, harmonizes the middle Jiao, and softens
  pain
~ Dispels cold, clears blood stagnation, and improves digestion

---

Indra makes footwear
that carries us from this world
on fragrant cushions

they are neither soft nor hard
but provide perfect support

I would burn my shoes
to perfume the heavens
with the wood from my soul

Wu Yao

Lindera Root
烏薬 (Uyaku)
Radix Linderae

Spicy, Warm
BL, KI, LU, SP

~ Promotes the movement of Qi, alleviates pain
~ Warms the kidneys and disperses cold

The friendly stallion
Letting go of the reins
it ran for the fence

I would have been excited
but I lost my grip on life

In my tai chi class
I get another chance
and enjoy the ride

Xiang Fu

Nut-Grass, Purple Nutsedge Root

香附 (Kobushi)

Rhizoma Cyperi

Slightly Bitter, Slightly Sweet, Spicy, Neutral
GB, LIV, TB,

~ Spreads and regulates liver Qi
~ Regulates menstruation alleviates pain

I once met a man:
little personality,
and was friends with all

Everyone likes listeners
except for other listeners

Proofreading my words
is infinity harder
then creating them

Xie Bai

Chives, Chinese Garlic
Bulbus Allii Macrostemi

Bitter, Spicy, Warm
LI, LU, ST

~ Unblocks the Yang Qi, clears turbidness, and disperses phlegm
~ Promotes the movement of Qi and Blood, alleviates pain, and
  disperses hardness
~ Directs Qi downward, reduces stagnation, and dries diarrhea

---

From the dim sum cart
we get single syllables
while others get names

25 visits later
we get an introduction

Yet when I bring guests
they assume I will translate
and call them by name

Zhi Ke

Bitter Orange
枳殼 (Kikoku)
Fructus Aurantii

Bitter, Spicy, Slightly Cold
SP, ST, LI

~ Moves Qi, reduce distention, eases pressure, and softens hardess

---

My high school heartthrob
a cynical girl
who wore orange underwear

it's like I knew a secret,
sunrise behind storm clouds

one time the day broke
and I said it wasn't bright
never saw the sun again

Zhi Shi

Unripe Bitter Orange

枳実 (Kijitsu)

Fructus Aurantii Immaturus

Bitter, Spicy, Cool
LI, SP, ST

~ Breaks up Qi stagnation, reduces accumulations, and transforms phlegm
~ Directs qi downward, removes stagnant food, and unblocks bowels.

No matter how fun
it only takes one asshole
to make things shitty

So we thought of the bouncer
who cut us off from more wine

Don't give me coffee
I just want to hear the song
of the cicada

Herbs That Anchor the Spirit

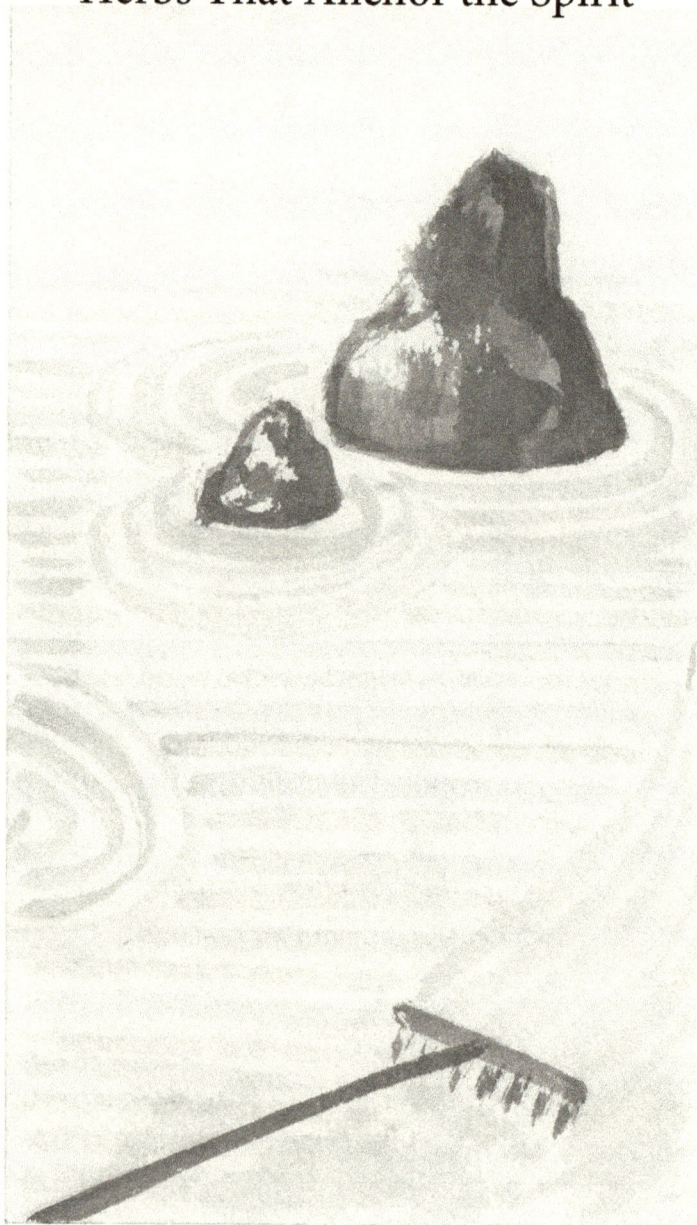

Ci Shi

Lodestone
Magnetitum

Spicy, Salty, Cold
KI, LIV

~ Anchors liver Yang and calms the spirit
~ Enrich the kidneys and liver
~ Helps kidneys to grasp Qi

Drawing all inward
Drawing up courage and strength
Drawing out true self

Place a lodestone in my heart,
I am attracted to you

Daylight's morning blade
made in Ise to cut through
the velvet of night

Hu Po

Amber

Succinum

Sweet, Neutral
BL, HRT, LIV

~ Stops tremors and palpitations, calm the spirit.
~ Invigorates the blood, dissipate stasis, and unblocks the menses.
~ Promotes and unblocks urination
~ Reduce swellings and promote healing

Ancient sap, tiger soul.
All fears departs the body
and falls to the ground.

The amber resin sutra
takes a million years to chant

No one sings that song
since the ancients converted
to builder's lumber

Long Gu and Long Qi

Dragon's Bones and Dragon's Teeth

竜骨 Ryukotsu

Fossilia Mastodi

Sweet, Astringent, Neutral
Long Gu: HRT, LIV, KI
Long Chi: HRT, LIV

~ Calms the spirit and eases anxiety
~ Calms the liver and anchors floating Yang
~ Prevents leakage of fluids due to deficiency
~ Topically for non-healing sores and ulcers.

Ancient teeth and bones
Transforms the timid rabbit
into a dragon

Did you hear about the carp?
He goes by the name Ryu

An old lady grinds
Her age becomes a number
Tiny to ancients

Mu Li

Oyster Shell
牡蠣 Borei
Concha Ostreae

Salty, Astringent, Cool
KI, LIV

~ Strongly anchors the spirit
~ Benefits the Yin, anchors floating Yang, and calms the liver
~ Prevents leakage of fluids
~ Absorbs acidity and pain in the stomach

A thousand sea shells
crash upon the soiled beach
and drag the filth down

The most humbles of cravings
A drop of the ocean's life

The shell cuts my lip
Salt mixes with blood and spit
I swallow the mess

Zhen Zhu

Pearl
Margarita

Sweet, Salty, Cold
HRT, LIV

~ Sedates the heart and calms tremor and palpitations.
~ Clears the liver and clears small visual obstructions.
~ Promotes healing and generates flesh.

Drops of purity
washes heat from the surface
of my skin and heart

The vain dissolve it in wine
Cannot undue what's been done

Sometimes it's the "truth"
of what we perceive as real
that clouds our vision

Zhu Sha

Cinnabar

Sweet, Cool, Very Toxic
HRT

~   Sedates the heart and calms the spirit
~   Clears phlegm and sedates nervous movement
~   Clears heat and resolves toxicity topically

Fool's Ruby
There is no life here
only death

Call out to Gogyo Yama
When the enemy rebels

Sometimes a mountain
can crush a great enemy
into a great friend

Bai Bian Dou

Hyacinth Bean
Semen Lablab Album

Sweet, Neutral to Slightly Warm
SP, ST

~ Clears summer heat and Dampness.
~ Strengthens the spleen
~ Treats overindulgence in food or alcohol

A night on the town
Filled with street food and liquor
Is nursed by a bean

I drink an extra bottle
Knowing at home, a nursemaid

Toilet bowel prayers;
I question my punishment
A beer tips over

He Ye

Lotus Leaf
Folium Nelumbinis

Bitter, Slightly Sweet, Neutral
HRT, LIV, SP

~ Treats summer heat
~ Raises and clears the spleen Yang, especially after summer heat
~ Stops bleeding in the lower Jiao

Upon the 8th leaf
Sits the Medicine Buddha
who lends you his chair

I ask you to clear my heat
I ask you to wrap my rice

Humbleness exists
when the flower is unplucked
and the leaf is pulled

Lu Dou

Mung Bean
Semen Phaseoli Radiati

Sweet, Cold
HRT, ST

~ Clears summer heat and quenches thirst.
~ Clears heat and toxins
~ Prevents overheating
~ Antidote to Fu Zi (Aconite).

A wise man once said
"Sprouted Mung Beans give me life,
but they smell like death"

If you care what you smell like
then your nose becomes your eyes

Sunny solitude
In a flower field I play
No one eats a skunk

Qing Hao

Sweet Wormwood

Artemisiae Annuae

Bitter, Cold
KI, LIV, GB

~ Clears summer heat
~ Clears blood or Yin deficient fever
~ Cools the blood and stops bleeding
~ Stops malarial disorders and clears liver heat

Pliny's bitter gift
"Health is an honorable prize"
Artemisiae

I see no yellow halo
and Van Gogh turns up his nose

Not all falling stars
signal the end of the world,
Perseid's herald

Xi Gua

Watermellon
Fructus Citrulli

Sweet, Bland, Cold
BL, HRT, ST

~ Clears summer heat and generates fluids
~ Promotes urination and removes jaundice
~ Cools lung and stomach heat

Under the noon sun
I bite the red flesh
and spit out the seeds

There is no manual labor
that Xi Gua cannot afford

My heart is grateful
Even my empty wallet
does not ask for more

Herbs That Clear Heat and Dry Dampness

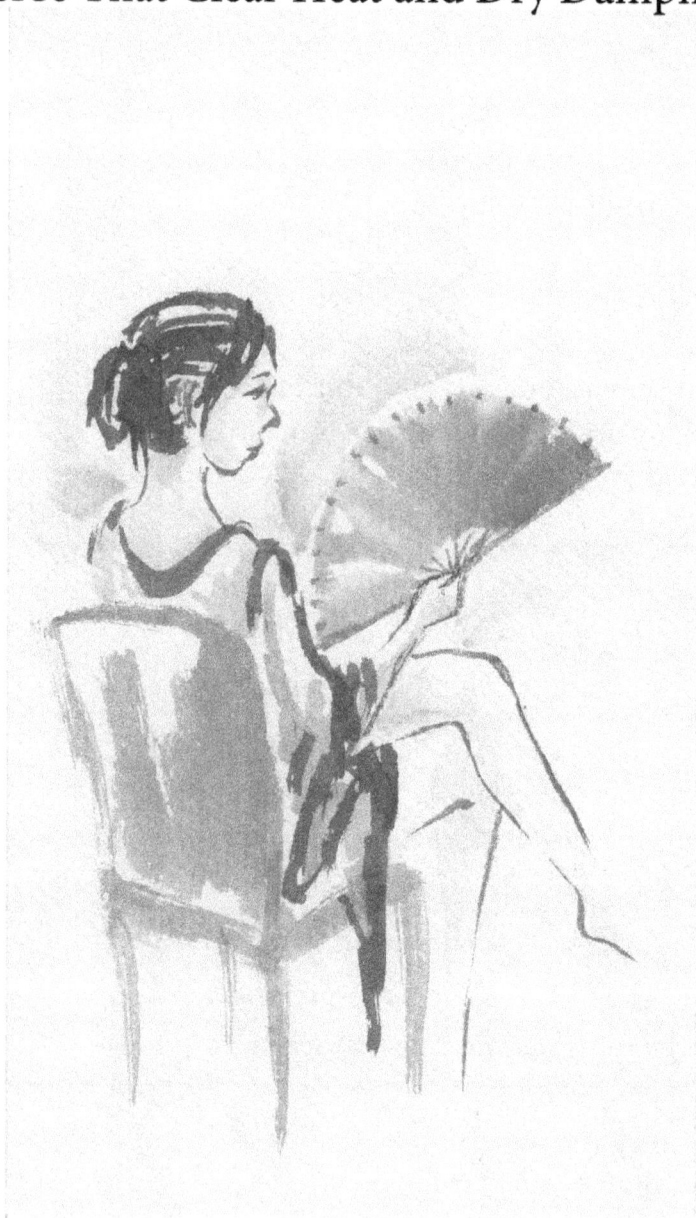

Huang Bai

Phellodendron Bark
黄柏 ōbaku
Cortex Phellodendri

Bitter, Cold
BL, KI

~ Drains damp heat in lower Jiao
~ Drains kidney Fire with kidney Yin deficiency
~ Drains Fire and heat toxicity
~ Can be toasted to decrease bitter and cold qualities

Ōbaku Bark.
For the thrifty and the wise
a panacea

Sometimes we reach for silver
when simple iron will do

A house built with wood
Moves with the wind and earthquake
while palaces fall

Huang Lian

Coptis Root
黃連 Ouren
Rhizoma Coptidis

Bitter, Cold
HRT, LI, LIV, ST

~ *Clears Heat and drains damp*
~ Drains Fire and related toxicities
~ Clears heat and stops bleeding
~ Calms heart and stomach fire

Cold and dry at heart,
yet grows in the damp and humid.
A Coloradan in Oregon

This land is much more fertile
for yucca and juniper

Ask Brother Yellow
when he finishes plowing
what crops you should sew

Huang Qin

Scute, Skullcap Root
黄芩 Ougon
Radix Scutellariae

Bitter, Cold
LU, ST, GB, LI

~ Clears heat and dries damp.
~ Drains fire and detoxifies
~ Clears heat and stops bleeding.
~ Clears heat and calms the fetus
~ Calms liver Yang rising

Yellow Aspirin,
your nine functions are hidden
behind bitter taste

A teacher shows discipline
Rigid reeds stand together

Merciless doctor
may leave a hole in my heart
but not in my chest

Ku Shen

Sophora, Pagoda Tree Root
苦参 Kujin
Radix Sophorae Flavescentis

Bitter, Cold
BL, HRT, LI, LIV, ST, SI

~ Clears heat and dries dampness
~ Kills parasites, stops wind and itching
~ Clears heat and promotes urination

Little Pagodas,
crafted by a master's hand
munched on by a cow

Masters build gifts to the world
The cow is just as grateful

At Kobo's Tō-ji
I remember meeting
a refreshing man

Long Dan Cao

Chinese Gentian Root
竜胆 Ryu Tan
Radix Gentianae

Bitter, Cold
GB, LIV, ST

~ Drains damp heat from the liver and gallbladder
~ Clears excessive liver fire

And you, looking up
with Azalea and Primula
The three king flowers

Hidden in the violet,
A fire-eating serpent

Purple ground dragon
Your gentleness bites my wrath
and drags it downward

Qin Pi

Korean Ash, Fraxinus Bark
Cortex Fraxini

Bitter, Astringent, Cold
GB, LI, LIV

~   Drains damp-heat
~   Drains liver fire
~   Clears wind-damp

Generous parents
The olive and the lilac
rear a kind child

A staff made of ask tree Bark
will support a lot of weight

To ones spitting flames
A patient man will listen;
extinguishing ears

Herbs That Clear Heat and Relieve Toxicity

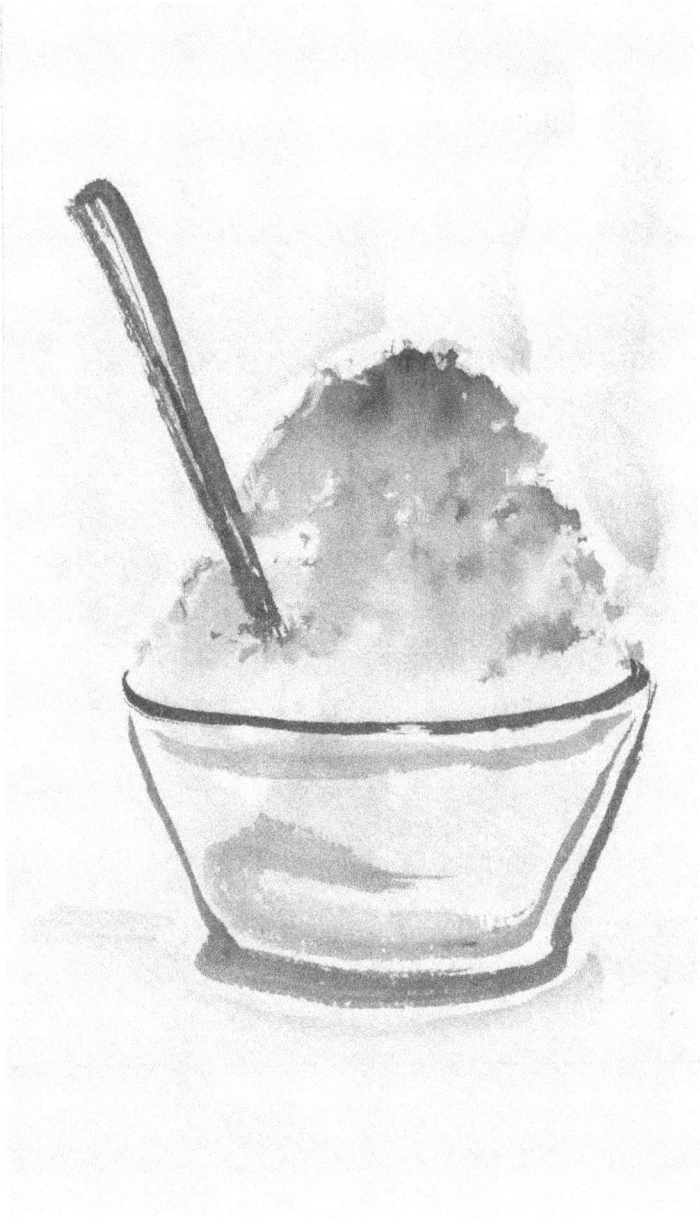

Bai Hua She She Cao

Hedyotis, Oldenlandia
Hedyotis Diffusae

Bitter, Sweet, Cold
LI, LIV, SI, ST

~ Clears heat, strongly relieve fire toxicity, reduces abscess
~ Clears heat and promotes urination

Awaiting his death
He mentions Oldenlandia
and sews seeds of life

His soul is made fireproof
on a hedyotis throne

Do you value herbs
more than the lives they save
Apothecary

Bai Tou Weng

Pulsatilla, Asian Pasqueflower Root
Radix Pulsatillae

Bitter, Cold
LI, ST

~ Clears heat and relieves fire toxicity
~ Stops fluid damage from heat
~ Good substitute for Goldenseal

In April we hunt
for what others have left us
painted and waiting

The purple Pulsatilla
Only serves sight in the west

No eggs left to find
And none left to be hidden
Empty nest syndrome

Bai Xing Pi

Chinese Dittany Root
Cortex Dictamn

Bitter, Cold
LI, ST

~ Clears heat and relieves fire toxicity
~ Expels wind and dries dampness
~ Clears damp heat and stops itching

In the Gas Plant's heart
is a tonic for the skin,
guarded by odor

The burning bush of the East
grows far from Moses' Horeb

A small cosmic joke,
that they could speak to Yahweh
through this stinking shrub

Ban Lan Gen

Isatis Root, Indigo Woad Root
Radix Isatis

Bitter, Cold
HRT, LU, ST

~ Drains heat and relieves fire toxicity
~ Cools the blood
~ Benefits the throat.
~ Grows in Colorado through Oregon

I always felt cool
in a sea of indigo.
Middle school denim

No one saw me in khaki
I stood out by blending in

I lost only fear
in my awkward camouflage
A lawn made of blades

Ban Zhi Lian

Bearded Scutellaria, Barbed Skullcap Root
Herba Scutellariae Barbatae

Spicy, Slightly Bitter, Cool
LIV, LU, ST

~ Clears heat, relieves fire toxicity
~ Invigorates the blood and reduces swelling
~ Reduces edema and promotes urination

I have a feeling
he would have shown us the herb
after the gallows

Knowledge does not disappear
It simply goes back to sleep

Cosmic library
I look through your card index
and long for Google

Chuan Xin Lian

Andrographis, Kalamegha
Andrographis paniculata

Bitter, Cold
LI, LU, SI, ST

~ Clears heat and relieves fire toxicity
~ Dries dampness and stops diarrhea
~ Cools the blood and resolves phlegm

Sometimes wisdom hides
in the bitter mouth of an ass
whispers in the brays

Slip some mint to the donkey
And let its yammers refresh

Who knows what burdens
Sapped the strength from the stallion
and broke the camel's back

Da Qing Ye

Indigo, Isatis Leaf
Folium Isatidis

Bitter, Salty, Very Cold, Slightly Toxic
HRT, LU, ST

~ Clears heat and relieves toxicity
~ Cools the blood and dissipates eruptions
~ Clears heart, lung, and stomach heat toxins

Once, at 3am
I broke out the clothing dye
Drunk in Tokyo

From the backyard bamboo grove
I call arashi shibori

Hyaka-en twine wrapped
Wikipedia tells me
How to make it rain

Hong Teng

Sargentodoxa Vine
Caulis Sargentodoxa

Bitter, Neutral
LI, LIV

~ Clears heat, relieves toxicity, and reduces abscesses
~ Invigorates the blood, stops pain, and disperses stasis

Only in the hills
do people know the secret
of the carved vine

Making wooden fetishes
from a pretty looking branch

I snap off an arm
And chew on it reverently
Medicine Buddha

Jin Yin Hua

Honeysuckle Flower, Woodbine
金銀花 (kinginka)
Flos Lonicerae

Sweet, Cold
LI, LU, ST

~   Clear heat, relieves fire toxicity
~   Expells wind heat
~   Clears damp heat from the lower Jiao

Innocent romance
Honeysuckle perfume
Spring is on a fling

The sweetness of a first date
cools his toxic bitterness

When a heart is burned
no ice can stop the damage
It still longs for fire

Lian Qiao

Forsythia Fruit
連翹, rengyo
Fructus Forsythiae

Bitter, Slightly Spicy, Slightly Cool
GB, HRT, LU

~ Clear heat and toxins in the upper Jiao
~ Reduces abscesses and swellings
~ Clears blood heat
~ Promotes urination

A golden bell rings
Apothecary aside
No one can hear it

I drink Lian Qlao tea
and my voice rings like a bell

We make harmony
With her sister, JIn Yin Hua
and sell it for a song

Ma Bo

Puffball
Lasiosphera

Spicy, Neutral
LU

~   Clears the lungs, relieves fire toxicity, and improves the throat
~   Topically to stop bleeding, especially around the mouth

Smoke from the lawn's egg
The Divine and his paintbrush
shows us his humor

We pluck miracles from dirt
And sauté them in butter

There is nothing wrong
Layers of miracles
Jawbreaker blessings

Ma Chi Xian

Purslane

Herba Portulacae

Sour, Cold
LI, LIV

~ Clears fire toxicity and cools the blood
~ Clears damp heat and treats sores
~ Antidote for wasp stings and snakebites.

It does not perish
when its uprooted and dried
A plant for pilgrims

Delicious in a salad
I follow the rabbits way

Like a pilgrimage
start slow and take a little
Joy builds with patience

Pu Gong Ying

Dandelion
蒲公英, hokoei
Herba Taraxac

Bitter, Sweet, Cold
LIV, ST

~ Clears heat, relieves fire toxicity, and unblocks urination
~ Dissipates nodules and reduces abscesses
~ Promotes lactation - due to heat.
~ Clears the liver and the eyes

Above emerald
a golden lion roaring
Common dandelion

They are not "Roundup Ready"
No one is "Roundup Ready"

Sometimes I'm the sun
Other times I am the moon
Either way, I bloom

Qing Dai

Processed Indigo Leaf
Indigo Naturalis

Salty, Cold
LIV, LU, ST

~ Cools the blood and reduces maculae
~ Clears heat and resolves fire toxicity
~ Drains liver fire and cools summer heat
~ Clears liver wind fire and lung heat

A cube of twilight
clears heat from the viscera
And washes the sky

Fires burn out in the night
Dark red cinders smoldering

He strikes wood on wood
"Beware of fires, beware!"
Mokuton alarm

Ren Dong Teng

Honeysuckle Vine Stem
忍冬, nindo
Caulis Lonicerae

Sweet, Cold
LI, LU, ST

~ Clears Heat and toxicity
~ Dispels wind dampness and unblocks the channels
~ Cools the blood
~ Clears damp heat from the lower Jiao
~ Expels wind heat

Deep in the rootstock
A sunset is blooming
to take away heat

Ignoring the twilight's horn
I look to solemn sources

From brown and woody
there is the slow seep of life
And all things spring forth

Shan Dou Gen

Bushy Sophora, Pigeon-Pea Root
Radix Sophorae Tonkinensis

Bitter, Cold, Slightly Toxic
LI, LU

~ Clears heat, relieves fire toxicity, improves throat
~ Clears damp heat jaundice

Garbage collector
Plucks leavings from the sidewalk
Feathered uniform

Someone called them "flying rats"
They need an AFSCME steward

Who could mistake them
What once was known as "Rock Dove"
is now detritus

She Gan

Blackberry Lilly Root
Rhizoma Belamcandae

Bitter, Cold
LU

~   Clears heat, relieves toxicity, and improves the throat
~   Transforms phlegm and clears the lungs

Did the leopard steal
The pattern from this lily,
or other way round

Maybe neither stole either
and both admired both?

Like the lily root
You diffuse my argument
and clear my fever

Tu Fu Ling

Smilax, Smooth Greenbriar Rhizome

土茯苓 (Dobukuryo)

Rhizoma Smilacis Glabre

Sweet, Bland, Neutral
LIV, ST

~ Relieves toxicity and clears dampness
~ Clears damp heat from the skin
~ Promotes urination and clears lower Jiao heat

Dark Age's treasure
Cousin of sarsaparilla
humble earthen root

Once precious in rarity
Now precious in your flavor

Essence of root beer
You quench my thirst and clear heat
One more, for the road

Tu Niu Xi

Tuniuxi Root

Radix Achryanthis Longae

Bitter, Sour, Neutral
LIV, KI

~ Drains fire and relieves toxicity
~ Clears heat toxin and heals abscesses and skin sores
~ Invigorates blood and dissipates stasis

Treasure of Ganesh,
Flower of two dozen names
You bring forth great change

You spur us to move faster
Devil's horsewhip at my feet

I don't have the heart
to use you in the way
a doctor could do

Ya Dan Zi

Bruceae Fruit

Fructus Bruceae

Bitter, Cold, Toxic

~ Clear heat and toxins, expels dampness, and cools the blood
~ Treats intermittent malarial disorders and kills parasites
~ Softens hardness

Ya Dan Zi
sounds like a New York waiter
asking "you done, sir?"

Rarely does a toxic plant
Sound as toxic as its name

It softens hardness
expels damp, cools the blood
And makes me giggle

Ye Ju Hua

Wild Chrysanthemum Flower
Flos Chrysanthemi Indici

Bitter, Spicy, Cool
LIV, LU

~   Drains fire and relieves toxicity

A barbarian,
tightly curled fists not blooming
Ye Ju Hua

A cousin claims refinement
Splayed out in garden troughs

A helpful neighbor
With an ear for your gossip
Flos chrysanthemi

Yu Xing Cao

Hottuynia, Fishwort Herb
Herba Hottuyniae

Spicy, Cool
LI, LU

~ Clears heat and toxins, reduces swellings and abscess
~ Relieves toxicity and expels pus for toxic sores
~ Drains damp-heat, promotes urination

A worn-down clinic
open late on a Friday.
Mud clam hides a pearl

Anointed badge of office;
Tongue depressors and lab coat

A doctor gives faith
by heating a stethoscope
with warm even breath

Zi Hua Di Ding

Violet, Earth Spike, Corydalis Bungeana
Herba Violae

Spicy, Bitter, Cold
HRT, LIV

~   Clears heat and fire toxicity
~   Clears hot sores internally and externally
~   Assists in the treatment of snakebite

The spike of the Earth
Steals venom from viper's fangs
and turns it to dirt

A bouquet of violets
take the sting out of her words

Nothing can stay hard
in the face of such softness
sumire yuri

Aromatic Herbs That Transform Dampness

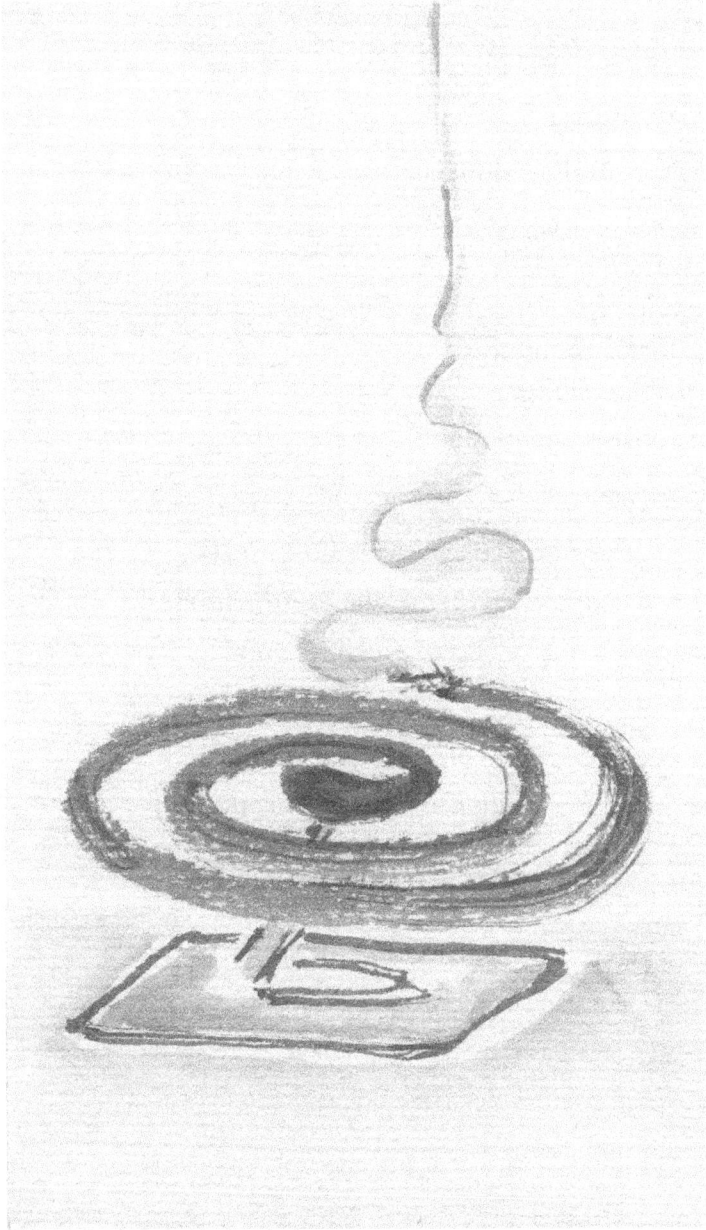

Bai Dou Kou

White Cardamom
Fructus Amomi Rotundus

Warm, Aromatic, Acrid
Lu, SP, ST

~ Transforms Dampness
~ Warms the middle
~ Transforms stagnation in the chest

Pungent smelling white
Soother of the middle jiao
greasy feelings gone

Father in the spice aisle
Matching mother's cooking

There is a flavor
That perfumes all of her food
Spiceless addition

Cang Zhu

Atractalodes

蒼朮 Sojutsu

Rhizoma Atractylodis

Spicy, Bitter, Warm, Aromatic
ST, ST

~ Strengthens Spleen and dries damp
~ Clears bi-syndrome in extremities.
~ Flushes damp-heat from lower burner

Herb like a bath robe;
warming, cooling, and drying
in the right places

Who puts on a big red robe
When all one needs is a sip

Smells like ripened cheese
From a land you can't visit
This woody rootstock

Cao Dou Kou

Grass Cardamom, Katsumada Galangal
Semen Alpiniae Katsumadai

Spicy, Warm, Aromatic
SP, ST

~ Dries dampness
~ Warms the middle burner
~ Strengthens the Spleen

Gently warms the spleen
distention and stomach woes
are carried away

What a name for piercing smell
"Wild grass cardamom pods"

Growing in the hills
Delightful discovery
Cherished by children

Cao Guo

Tsaoko Fruit
Fructus Amomi Tsaoko

Spicy, Aromatic, Warm
SP, ST

~ Strongly dries dampness and warms the middle Jiao
~ Relives malarial symptoms
~ Dissipates heat stagnation, distention, and phlegm

Pearls from the Devil.
A gift that overcomes cold
with a smell like hell

Embers in a fireplace
Makes ice water look like tea

A smoky fire
Drives away the mosquitos
Drives in the campers

Hou Po

Magnolia Bark
厚朴 Kobuku
Cortex Magnoliae Officinalis

Bitter, Spicy, Aromatic, Warm
LI, LU, SP, ST

~ Resolves stagnation of Qi in the Middle Jiao
~ Transforms phlegm and dries Damp.
~ Descends Rebellious Qi

In the waxy green
are flowers white like heaven
but smell like brimstone

Amethysts and ivory
I bring to you in bunches

I think of the South
A place I have never been,
Outside of airports

Pei Lan

Orchid Grass
Herba Eupatorii

Spicy, Neutral, Slightly Toxic
SP, ST

~ Transforms Damp and awakens the Spleen.
~ Clears early summer heat and transforms damp.
~ Clears turbidity in the middle Jiao

I seek relief from
the rain of the summer sun
in sheaves of tall grass

Filed away from the heat
I sit inside, looking out

In the summer we beg
for the relief we curse
throughout the winter

Sha Ren

Cardamom, Grains of Paradise
縮砂 (砂仁) Shukusha
Fructus Amomi

Spicy, Aromatic, Warm
SP, ST

~ Moves Qi, Transforms Damp, Strengthens Spleen, and stops vomiting.
~ Warms the middle, Stops Diarrhea.
~ Prevents tonifying herbs from causing stagnation

Bright transforming herb
excites the middle Jiao
and calm the unborn

Moderating indulgence
it keeps the party going

Guarding stomach's bar
the aromatic bouncer;
Grains of paradise

Huo Xiang

Patchouli
藿香 Kakko
Herba Agastaches

Spicy, Aromatic, slightly warm
LU, SP, ST

~ Dispels dampness, opens the doors, and relieves summer heat
~ Harmonizes the Middle Jiao and eases vomiting.
~ Treats fungal infections of the hands and feet.

A hippie's blessing:
Relief from the sun sickness,
nausea, and fungus

In a yellow Vanagon
I see specters of the past

Hitching on bumpers
manifold aspirations
On sticky paper

Herbs For External Applications

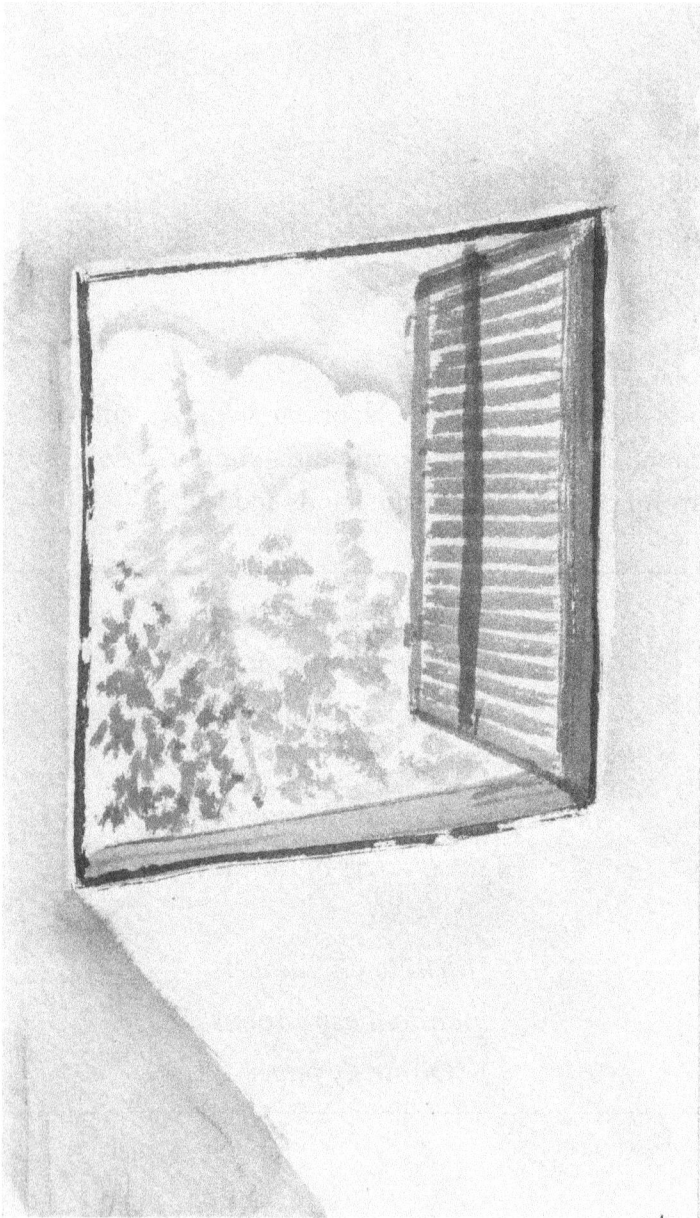

Ban Mao

Chinese Blister Beetle
斑猫 Hanmyo
Mylabris

Spicy, Cold, Very Toxic
LI, LIV, SI

~ Attack toxins and softens sores
~ Breaks apart clumps and blood stasis
~ Causes blistering and strong movement on the skin

A pain for everyone
that gives hope to many.
What a humble bug

Barefoot step on Hanmyo
reminds me that life is short

Phobia of death
Makes us shut our eyes to life,
Drives people to pain

Liu Huang

Sulphur

Sour, Hot, Toxic
KI, LI, PER

~ Relieves toxicity, kills parasites, stops itching.
~ Tonifies MingMen fire and strengthen Yang

The smell of yellow
The smell of burnt earth and springs
The smell of healing

Only one sense is needed
To find healing waters

Sharp smell makes me ask
"industry or history?"
My nose rejects both

Lu Feng Fang

Wasp Nest
Nidus Vespae

Sweet, Neutral, Toxic
LU, ST

~ Relieve toxicity, expel wind, relieves itching and pain.
~ Expel wind and dries dampness
~ Treats tumors and parasites

Driving out wind,
this home to yellowjackets
is most inviting.

A fear of occupation
leads to turbid residents

Creatures smelling fear
Sedged-hat in Tokyo
Draw their knives and shout

Lu Gan Shi

Calamine

Smithsonitum

Sweet, Neutral
LIV, ST

~ Brightens the eyes
~ Dries dampness and generates flesh
~ Stops itching and resolves toxicity

You cut short the grip
when poison ivy grabbed me
with its burning grasp

Moonlight on the bathroom floor
I wait for the mud to dry

Covered in the pink
I regret my careless joy
and its ceaseless itch

Ma Qian Zi

Nux Vomica, Horse Money Seeds
Semen Strychnotis

Bitter, Cold, Very Toxic
LIV, SP

~ Unblocks the channels and disperse clumps
~ Reduces swelling and alleviates pain.
~ Cools blood heat

One incurs a debt
when paying in Horse Money.
Can you foot the bill?

If there is no bill to foot
If is my feet that will pay

In western markets
To go up you must go down
The cycle of debt

Ming Fan

Alum

Sour, Astringent, Cold
LI, LIV, LU, SP, ST

~ Relieves toxicity, kills parasites, dry dampness, alleviate itch.
~ Generates flesh and transforms putrid stagnation.
~ Stops bleeding and lessens diarrhea
~ Clears heat and expels phlegm

Friend of the Romans,
Who used you to clean water
And save shaved faces

My aunt's kitchen, long ago
The alum tin gathers dust

Next to the allspice
You were regrettably bland
And never sold well

Qing Fen

Mercury

Calomelas

Spicy, Cold, Very Toxic
BL, KI, LIV

~ Kills parasites and promotes the healing of sores.
~ Expels water and unblocks the bowels and bladder.

Oh Lewis and Clark.
They, who took Rush's Thunder,
left echoing pits.

Of heroic medicine
I only trust history

Loving intention:
Even paper becomes pills,
And poison cures pain

She Chuang Zi

Cnidium Seeds

蛇床子 Jashoshi

Fructus Cnidii Monnieni

Spicy, Bitter, Warm, Slightly Toxic
KI, SP

~ Dry dampness, kills parasites, stop itching on the skin
~ Warms the kidneys and strengthens yang
~ Disperses cold and wind

Hide with me under
A delicate umbrella
And I'll heal your wounds

You can't protect from the rain
While watching out for serpents

Only drunkards share
In the leaves of "Jashoshi"
A bed made for snakes

Xiong Huang

Arsenic Sulfide

Realgar

Spicy, Bitter, Warm, Very Toxic
HT, LIV, ST

~   Relieves toxicity and kills parasites

Only ghosts are made
when "Masculine Yellow"
Is mixed into wine

In a world full of bounty
who would eat bitter parts?

Sharp shell hides the yolk
Rind holds the watermelon
Parsley tops carrots

Herbs That Cool and Transform Phlegm Heat

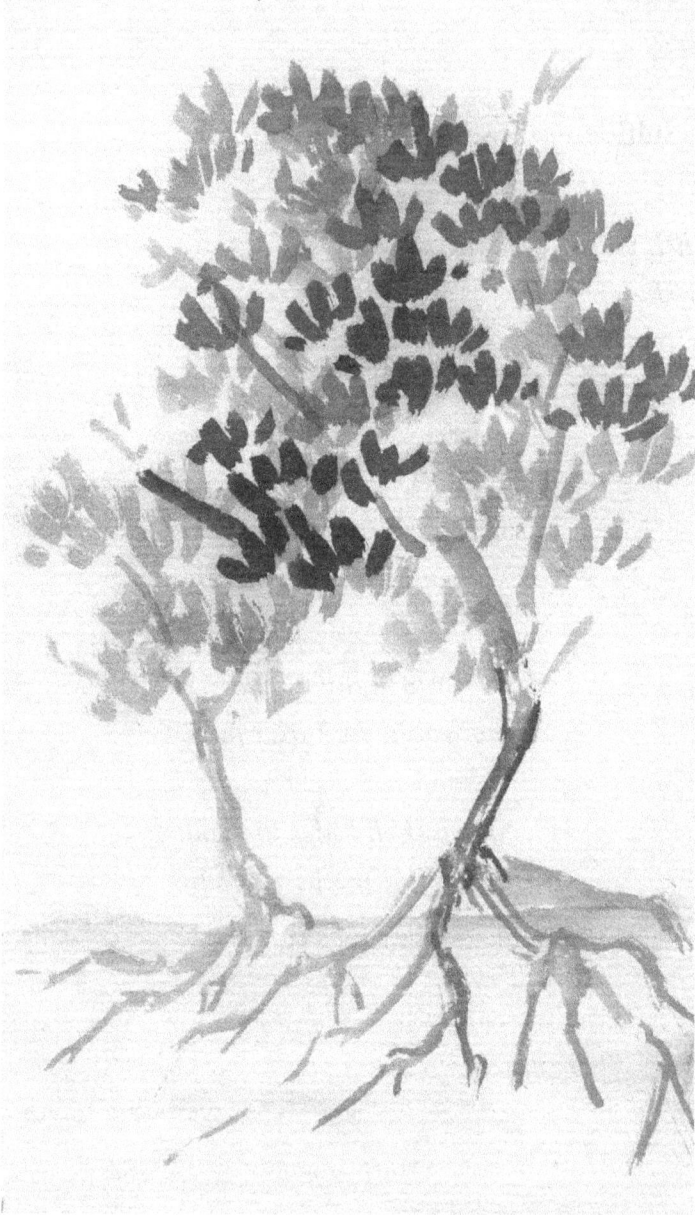

Chuan Bei Mu

Fritillaria Bulb
Bulbus Fritillariae Cirrhosae

Bitter, Sweet, Cool
HRT, LU

~ Clears heat, transforms phlegm, stops coughing, and moistens the lungs
~ Clears heat and dissipates heat-related nodules
~ Directs heart fire downward

A mother's first time
She guides a gift towards her mouth
and prays for abundance

Grandma give her Chuan Bei Mu
Tears and milk both start flowing

What was given to her
from breast to mouth
for eternity

Dan Nan Xing

Arisaemae in bile
Pulvis Arisaemae cum Felle Bovis

Bitter, Cool, Slightly Toxic
LIV, LU, SP

~   Transforms phlegm heat extinguishes wind, stops convulsions

---

Bitter on bitter
What did I do to deserve this
Bitter on bitter

I tremor at the odor
and I tremor without it

Convulsing, I drink
Gagging, I hold the black down
Resting, I'm thankful

Fu Hai Shi

Costaziae Skeleton, White Pumice
Os Costaziae

Salty, Cold
LU

~ Clears heat from the lungs and removes phlegm
~ Softens hardness and dissipates phlegm nodules
~ Promotes urination and unblocks the lungs

Aquatic wormstone
Float on the sea stone
Who found health in you?

No one looked at river mud
and saw the gold in the silt

Yet who could deny
that a stone that does not sink
is less than magic

Gua Lou

Snakegourd Fruit
Fructus Trichosanthis

Sweet, Cold
LI, LU, ST

~ Clears heat and transforms hot phlegm
~ Reduces abscesses and dissipates nodules
~ Regulates and loosens Qi in the chest

Geisha of Basho
Closed petals during the day
Loose lace at night

Cold blooded, they steal my warmth
And open up when I cool

When the bud falls off
what was a delicate bloom
becomes nourishment

Gua Lou Ren

Snakegourd Seed(Karonin)

栝楼仁 (Karonin)

Semen Trichosanthis

Sweet, Cold
LIV, LU, ST

~ Clears heat and transforms phlegm
~ Expands the chest.
~ Moistens the intestines
~ Assists other herbs in expelling pus and promoting healing of
  sores

The Geisha's Sunday;
Repairing her kimono,
Drinking guava juice

She stores her painted smile
and chooses what face to wear

Hair down, now common
Her workplace giggle slips though
in the checkout line

Hai Ge Ke/ Ge Qiao

Clam Shell

Concha Cyclinae / Concha Meretricis

Bitter, Salty, Cold
LU, ST

~ Clears lung heat, descends lung qi, transforms phlegm
~ Softens hardness and dissipates nodules
~ Promotes urination and expels turbid dampness
~ Eases pain due to stomach acid and heat.

I dreamed my foot caught
in the bite of a clam shell
tangled in bedsheets

Unreasonable phobia
keeps me from diving too deep

Will my shell be used
As an herbal remedy
for a giant clam?

Hai Zao

Sargassum Seaweed
Herba Sargassii

Bitter, Salty, Cold
Ki, LIV, LU, ST

~ Clears heat, reduces phlegm, and softens hardness
~ Helps promote urination and reduces edema

Looking at her hands
Volcanoes and Sargasso
The hula dance

The I'pu 'pu thumping
Pele's children and twirling

Under a white tent
Her shining eyes, orchid lay
Hula wedding dance

Huang Yao Zi

Potato Yam Tuber

Rhizoma Dioscoreae Bulbiferae

Bitter, Cold
LIV, LU

~ Dissipates nodules, clears phlegm, and reduces masses
~ Cools the blood and stops bleeding
~ Clears heat and reduces toxicity (surface and internally)

Climbing up a pole
I wonder what will happen
when the vine connects

The climbing root does not care
if it grounds the power line

Hanging from a line
A curious gourd peeks through
A tuber dangles

Kun Bu

Kelp, Japanese Sea Tangle
Thallus Eckloniae
Salty, Cold
KI, LIV, ST

~ Reduces phlegm and softens nodules
~ Promotes urination and reduces swelling.

Faithful companion
Always lapping at my feet
Pacific ocean

Today it brings me a shell
Tomorrow, an octopus

A bottled message
Ocean waves playing fetch with
my future version

Pang Da Hai

Sterculia Seed

Semen Sterculiae Lychnophorae

Sweet, Cold
LI, LU

~ Clears and disseminates lung Qi
~ Moistens the intestines and unblocks the bowels
~ Helps encourage the expression of rashes

Approaching the stage
He belts out a song and says
"it's gonna be ok"

Friday night karaoke
Broken hearts and dollar beer

Bowery bird barfly
Displaying blue tinted songs
Looking for a mate

Qian Hu

Asian Masterwort Root, Hogfennel
Radix Peucedani

Bitter, Spicy, Cool
LU

~ Moves rebellious lung qi downward and clears phlegm
~ Clears wind-heat from the exterior and loosens the lungs

Four wild black hogs
at a quick clip down the road
Escape hungry eyes

In a land of poverty
do ancient morals fill you?

Bacon and freedom
Given with good intentions
on a gun's barrel

Gua Luo Gen / Tien Hua Fen

Snakegourd Root

栝楼根 (karokon)

Radix Trichosanthis

Bitter, Slightly Sweet, Cold
LU, ST

~ Clears and drains lung heat, transforms phlegm, and moistens
   lung dryness.
~ Drains heat and generates fluid
~ Relieves toxicity, reduces swelling, and expels pus

In our paradise
the root is where the snake lives
Striking when eyes stray

A bite that doesn't hurt
Cooling, draining, relieving

Aches like a venom
We look for a remedy
in a pair of fangs

Tian Zhu Huang

Tabasheer, Bamboo Sugar
Concretio Bambusae Silicea

Sweet, Cold
GB, HRT, LIV

~ Clears and transforms phlegm heat
~ Clears heat, cools the heart, and calms tremors

Fingers of the Earth
I crack your knuckles loudly
and borrow your marrow

How can you borrow something
when you cannot replace it?

A loan between friends
should be considered a gift
that celebrates love

Zhe Bei Mu

Zhejian Fritillaria Bulb
Bulbus Fritillariae Thunbergii

Bitter, Cold
HRT, LU

~ Clears and transforms phlegm heat
~ Stops cough
~ Clears heat and dissipates nodules

Its famous brother
Gets all attention
This, behind the scenes

A stagehand; the gatekeeper
The spotlight worker, the sun

The cousins perform
Zhejian, the somber actor
Fritillaria

Zhu Ru

Bamboo Shavings
竹筎 (chikujo)
Caulis Bambusae in Taeniam

Sweet, Cool
LU, ST

~ Clears and transforms phlegm heat
~ Clears heat from the stomach and stops vomiting
~ Cools the blood and stops bleeding

Walking in the grove
Sound of bamboo applauding
The way home, closed

Expanding and contracting
Cobwebs in the forest lungs

Once, in Kyoto
A hummingbird followed me
Nope, a honey wasp

Herbs That Cool the Blood

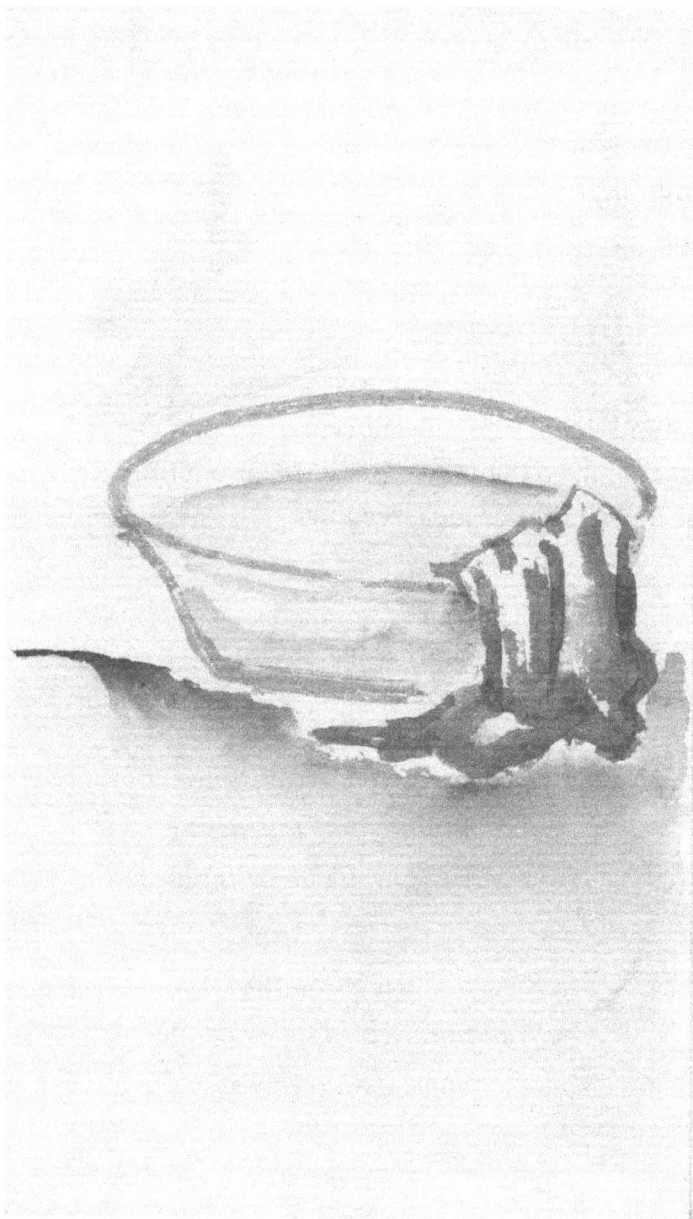

Bai Wei

Swallowwort Root

Radix Cynachi Atrati

Bitter, Salty, Cold
KI, LU, ST

~ Clears deficient heat and cools blood
~ Promotes urination
~ Relieves toxicity and toxic sores

Black drops plummeting
Swallows dive bomb from rooftops
My dog and I watch

She came to me in a dream
And offered me her fur coat

For want of a ball
and a scratch behind the ears
she gives me her heart

Di Gu Pi

Wolfberry Root, Lycium Root
地骨皮 (jikoppi)
Cortex Lycii

Sweet, Bland, Cold
Ki, LIV, LU

~ Drains Yin deficiency fire and eliminates lurking heat.
~ Clears lung heat.
~ Clears heat, cools blood, and stops bleeding

Marble and ivy
Fujin and Raijin of books
Library columns

One supporting, one binding
Stitching together a book

For a streak-free shine
vinegar and newspaper
The diamond clear mind

Mu Dan Pi

Tree Peony Root Bark

牡丹皮 (botanpi)

Cortex Moutan

Spicy, Bitter, Cool
HRT, KI, LIV

~ Clears both excess and deficient heat and cools blood
~ Clear deficient fire
~ Clears liver blood stasis and clears liver fire
~ Drains pus and reduces swelling

Cut into slices
your peel look like snail shells
Oh, tree Peony

Cooling and grounding
Liquid granite decoction

Skin of the mountain
Even if grown on the plains
you taste like the foothills

Sheng Di Huang

Chinese Foxglove Root
地黄 (Jio)
Radix Rehmanniae

Sweet, Bitter, Cold
HRT, KI, LIV

~ Clears Heat and cools the blood.
~ Nourishes Yin and generates fluids.
~ Cools ascending heart fire.

Sticky and secret
the taste of the fox glove root
is the taste of Yin

When in bloom, my heart stops
When looks fade, my heart beats stronger

With ill intentions
no one should pull up the root;
A cloying sweetness

Xi Jiao

Rhinoceros Horn
犀角 (saikaku)
Cornu Rhinoceri

Bitter, Salty, Cold
HRT, LIV, ST

~ Clears deep stage heat and fire toxicity
~ Clears the heart and calms the Shen
~ Extinguishes liver wind and heat

There is no drug here
Just the poison of money
and a horn of hair

Feral pigs gnaw at false bone
and dream of being human

A poacher is shot
I mourn his situation
but not much else

Xuan Shen

Ningpo Figwort Root
Radix Scrophulariae

Salty, Sweet, Bitter, Cold
KI, LU, ST

- ~ Clears heat and cools blood
- ~ Nourishes Yin.
- ~ Drains fire and relieves toxicity.
- ~ Softens hardness and dissipates hot nodules.

The autumn harvest
Digging up the plant's lowers
to treat our uppers

Ill, I croak like a bullfrog
My neck swelling outward

Fields going fallow
How many adventures die
while I sit on the couch

Yin Chai Hu

Starwort Root

Radix Stellariae

Sweet, Cool
LIV, ST

~ Clears deficient heat
~ Helps ease symptoms related to childhood nutritional impairment due to heat accumulation
~ Cools blood, and stops bleeding.

The candy aisle
A child begs for a treat
Mom acquiesces

Praying for jelly bean rain
and chocolate coin riches

Don't lose that eye glint
to the dullness of the world
Oh my darling girl

Zi Cao

Groomwell Root, Chinese Stoneseed
Radix Lithopermi, Radix Arnbiae

Sweet, Cold
HRT, LIV

~ Clears heat, cools the blood, relieves fire toxicity and encourages
  the expression of rashes.
~ Clears damp heat from the skin
~ Moisten the intestines and unblock the bowels.

One is soft purple herb
hiding below its flowers
One is hard purple herb

Brother to borage and comfrey
You come from good roots

They hide their beauty secret
in pearls filled with clear oil
Nobless oblige

Herbs That Dispel Wind Dampness

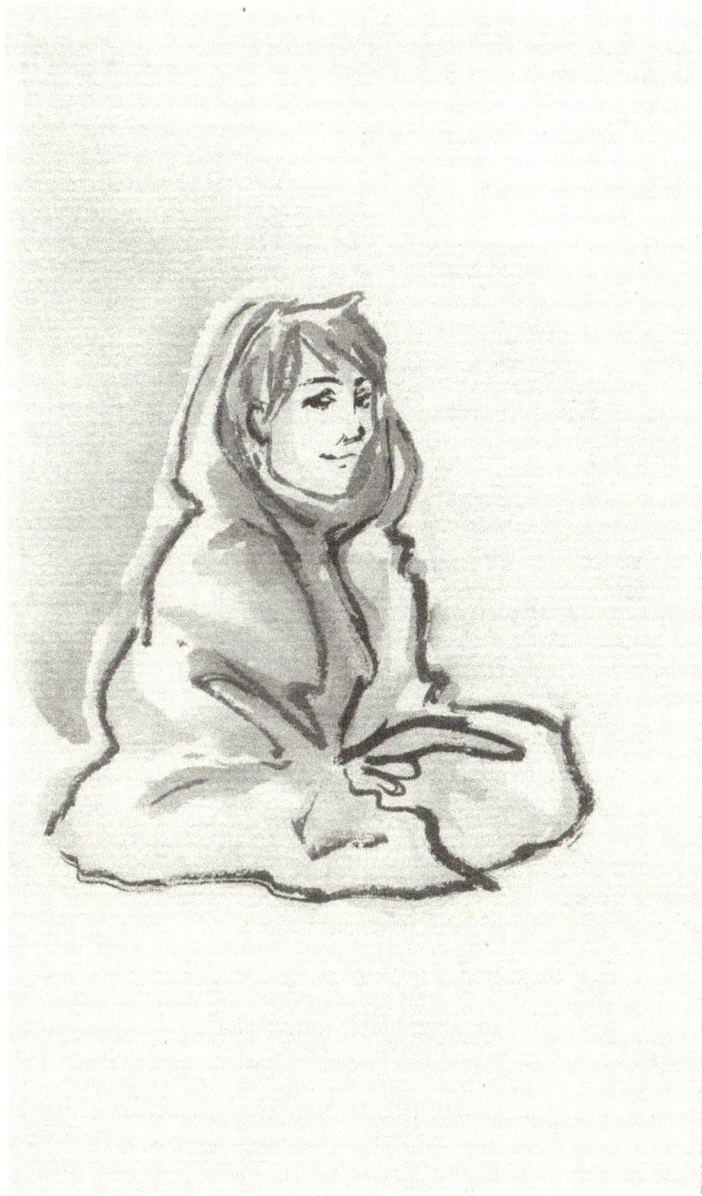

Bai Hua She / Qi She

Banded Krait, White Flower Snake

Agkistrodon / Bungarus

Salty, Sweet, Warm Toxic
LIV

~ Powerfully unblocks the channels and dispels wind.
~ Extinguishes wind from the skin and sinews and settles convulsions.

Blocking many hits
I wrap my wrists in vipers
and keep on fighting

That with the greatest venom
is also the most timid

The rattlesnake lies
buzzing with mock lethalness
The krait carries death

Can Sha

Silkworm Feces

Excrementum Bombycis Mori

Spicy, Sweet, Warm
LIV, SP, ST

~ Expels wind and dampness
~ Harmonizes the stomach and transforms turbid dampness

In the most skilled hands
even shit becomes treasure
Silkworm excrement

Royalty wear the moltings
of those which overcame themselves

Casting off treasure
My soul goes flying freely
to feed on nectar

Cang Er Zi

Cocklebur Fruit, Xanthium Fruit
Fructus Xanthii

Sweet, Bitter, Warm, Toxic
LU

~ Expels wind dampness and opens the sinuses
~ Dispels exterior wind and dampness

So anxious to help
it hitches to my clothing
and invites itself home

Toyama no kusuri
No one likes your sales pitch

Oh Baiyaku-san
was this job always your dream?
Can't sell oil now

Du Huo

Pubescent Angelica Root

Radix Angelicae Pubenscentis

Bitter, Spicy, Warm
BL, KI

~ Dispels wind cold damp and releases the exterior.
~ Dispels wind dampness and alleviates pain
~ Treats Shao Yin level headache and toothache.

There is a sweetness
that changes to bitter spice
late in the springtime

What once was of the rootstock
Severs its parental bond

The canes, once weeping
branch out and reach for the sun
Their very own sun

Hai Feng Teng

Kadsura Pepper Stem, Futokadsura Stem
Caulis Piperis Kadsurae

Spicy, Bitter, Slightly Warm
LIV

~ Dispels wind dampness bi and opens the channels.
~ Disperses cold and alleviates pain

A link without hands
Before the Kanmon tunnel
Futokadsura

Ruby pendent drupes
Jewelry from Ryukyu

Seeing drops of home
Back straightens, cold disappears
nostalgia medicine

Hai Tong Pi

Erythina Bark, Coral-Bean Bark
Cortex Erythrinae

Bitter, Spicy, Neutral
KI, LIV, SP

~ Dispels wind damp (hot or cold) and unblocks the channels.
~ Promotes urination and reduces edema
~ Treats itchy skin lesions and kills parasites
~ Soothes toothache due to cavities

A fire burning
Without scorching the soil
or burning my nose

The parasites are foolish
and run screaming from the "flames"

Plant this at your root
let it drive off the dampness
that chills in your heart

Luo Shi Teng

Star Jasmine Stem
Caulis Trachelospermi

Bitter, Cool
LIV

~ Dispels wind damp heat while opening the channels and
  collaterals
~ Cools the blood and reduces swelling.

Behind the factory
Cascading over the wall
fragrant abundance

All winter, a skeleton
All summer, a thing of flesh

For just a few days
the white hard-hats come off,
noses turn skyward

Mu Gua

Chinese Quince Fruit
木瓜 (Mokka)
Fructus Chaenomelis

Sour, Warm
LIV, SP

~ Relaxes the sinews and muscles and unblocks the channels.
~ Harmonizes the stomach, transforms dampness, reduces food stagnation, and nourishes the liver

---

Deep in forest park
Looking, bending, and stashing
I harvest the quince

Arboretum charity
Wood giving alms to the poor

Like a Fruit ninja
not a leaf or branch tremors
Fruit disappears

Qin Jiao

Large-Leaf Gentiana Root, Chin-Chiu

Radix Gentianae Macrophyllae

Bitter, Spicy, Slightly Cold
GB, LIV, ST

~ Expels Wind-Dampness, opens the channels, and soothes the sinews and collaterals
~ Clears deficient heat
~ Alleviates jaundice and resolves dampness.
~ Moistens the intestines and bowels

Wrapped up in softness
I can let go of evil
The way a child can

Even when the cat scratches
She strokes with a steady hand

Involuntary
It's in its nature to strike
and in hers to tame

Sang Zhi

Mulberry Twig
Ramulus Mori

Bitter, Neutral
LIV

~ Clears wind dampness, unblocks the channels and collaterals,
  helps the joints and stops spasms.
~ Reduces edema and promotes urination.

Caterpillar road
Your branches give directions
to a leafy home

Such a generous city
to both guests and residents

I harvest the Fruit
and feed the butterfly
in my fleeting dream

Wei Ling Xian

Chinese Clematis Root
威霊仙 (ireisen)
Radix Clematidis

Salty, Spicy, Warm, (some consider Toxic)
BL

~ Dispels wind damp, unblocks the channels, and relieves pain.
~ Softens fish bones lodged in the throat.
~ Reduces distention in the middle Jiao

Desperate for flavor
They carried clematis seeds
and called them pepper

If hard tack was my supper
I'd eat dirt and call it salt

Exorcising tea
A ghost swimming upstream
fishbone in my throat

Wu Jia Pi

Siberian Ginseng, Eleuthrococcus Root,
五加皮 (gokahi)
Cortex Acanthopanacis

Bitter, Spicy, Warm
KI, LIV

~ Dispels wind damp, strengthens the sinews and bones, nourishes the liver and kidneys
~ Transforms dampness and reduces swelling

Mistaken for Red
From the land of the Reds
Five Additions Root

Banished to Siberia
for being poorly marketed

With a heart of white
it should travel everywhere
I grant a visa

Wu Shao She

Black Grass Snake
Zaocys, Coulbridae

Salty, Sweet, Neutral
LIV, SP

~ Strongly unblocks the channels and extinguishes Wind
~ Dispels wind from the skin
~ Dispels wind from the sinews, strengthens tendons and bones, and settles jitteriness

---

Some judge the black snake, thin as paper
Against all serpentkind
Yet it does not strike

Not all that is black is night
Not all vipers have venom

Fangless or barbed
I still fear being bitten
By the rope of dark

Xi Xian Cao

St. Paul's Wort, Siegesbeckiae
Herba Siegesbeckia

Bitter, Cold
KI, LIV

~ Dispels wind damp heat, strengthens the sinews, and unblocks the channels
~ Calms the spirit, clears heat, and pacifies the liver
~ Clears toxins and transforms damp heat

"Loathsome Harlotry"
Such strong words were once spoken
regarding naming

It is truly ironic
That his name is now an herb

Perhaps as a plant
He'll enjoy "harlotry"
that he once denied

Herbs That Drain Dampness

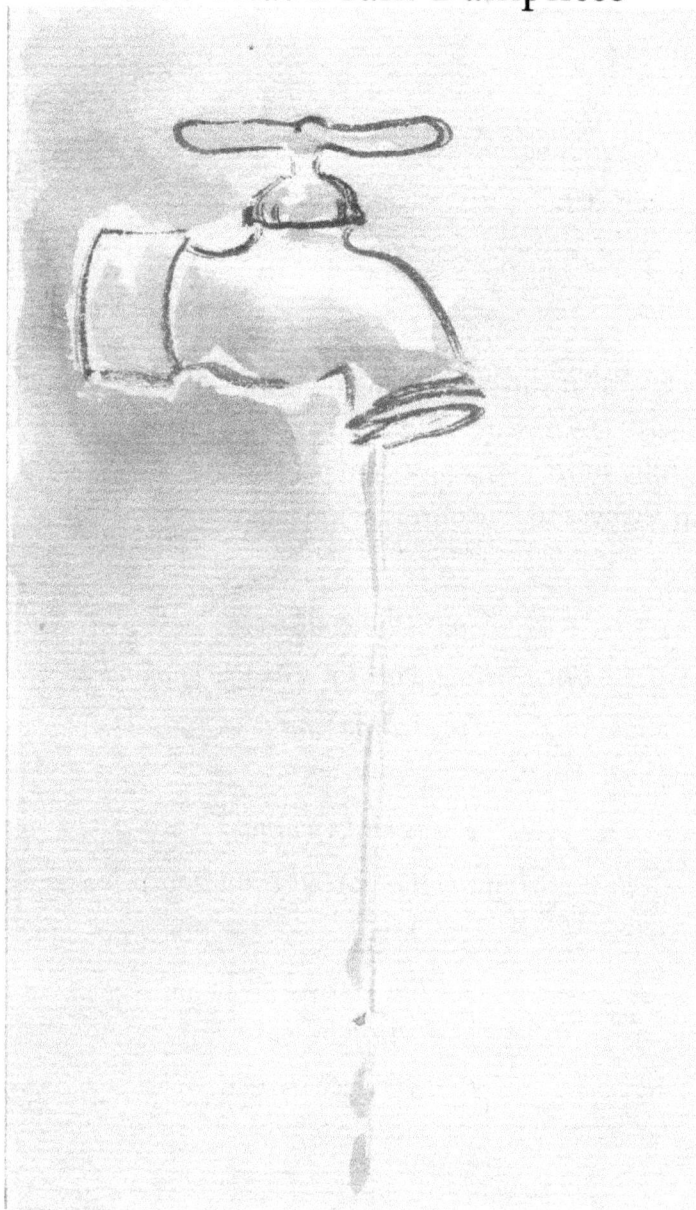

Ban Bian Lian

Chinese Lobelia
Herba Lobeliae Chinensis

Sweet, Bland, Slightly Cold
HRT, SI, LU

~ Promotes urination and reduces edema
~ Cools the blood, clears heat, and reduces toxicity

She chews on the leaf
and then spat the green wad out
on grandson's bee sting

in the world of microscopes
no one can trust abuela

her knowledge fading
it returns to the soil
from which it once came

Bei Xie

Tokoro, Fish Poison Yam Rhizome
Rhizoma Dioscoreae Hypoglaucae

Bitter, Neutral
BL, LIV, ST

~ Separates the pure from the turbid in the lower Jiao
~ Expels wind damp, relaxes sinew, and unblocks the channels
~ Clears damp heat from the skin

Slice a potato
and throw it in the water
All the fish float up

Is there cheating in fishing?
If there is, please show me how

There is no honor
in going to bed hungry
Calorie-free pride

Bian Xu

Polygonum, Knotweet
Herba Polygoni Avicularis

Bitter, Slightly Cold
BL

~ Clears damp heat from the bladder
~ Expels parasites and stops itching.

Knotweed history
twisted roots grow straight flowers
Past choking present

I will tie my heart in knots
and you can untangle me

I cannot unbind
with my roots knotted too,
I'll trust into you

Che Qian Zi

Asian Plantain Seeds
車前子 (shazenshi)
Semen Plantaginis

Sweet, Cold,
BL, KI, LI, LU

~ Promotes urination and clears heat
~ Solidifies the stool and promotes urination.
~ Clears Liver Heat and clears the eyes
~ Clears the lungs, expels phlegm, and stops cough.

Barefoot in the thorns
my father shows me plantain
and I never forgot

on his back we crosses the weeds
poison ivy brushing ankles

Brother got it worse
He tried to tread on a path
not revealed to him

Chi Xiao Dou

Aduki Bean
Semen Phaseoli

Sweet, Sour, Neutral
HRT, SI

~ Clears heat, promotes urination, and reduces edema,
~ Disperses blood stasis, swelling, and fire toxicity
~ Clears damp heat and jaundice.

Outside the temple
Obasan shares her spirit
red beam buns

her hands work without thinking,
heart connected to her wrist

there's no recipe
only scoops and pinches
from unlabeled tins

Deng Xin Cao

Bulrush Pith
Medulla Junci

Sweet, Bland, Slightly Cold
HRT, LU, SI

~ Promotes urination, draws out dampness, unblock urinary
  function
~ Clears heat from the heart channel into the small intestine and
  calms the spirit

"A drink between friends"
is what we call the third
the first, a business meeting

We sometimes drown our sadness
in a happy pint-size bath

It hangs from my heart
Resisting the waterslide
Leading to paradise

Di Fu Zi

Broom Cypress, Belvedere Fruit
Fructus Kochiae

Sweet, Bitter, Cold
BL, KI

~ Clears damp heat and promotes urination
~ Expels dampness and stops itching
~ Clears wind heat affecting the head

After collapse
the brave and the poor return
Urban pioneer

Deep in the auto city
Corn stalks peek over bumpers

A decade of change
for the lone cartographer
Google Maps archive

Dong Gua Zi

Winter Mellon Seed, Wax Gourd Seed
冬瓜子 (togashi)
Semen Benincasae

Sweet, Cold
LU, LI, SI, ST

~ Clears lung and intestinal heat, expels phlegm, clears pus, and moistens the lungs
~ Clears heat and drains dampness

The frost upon frost
Honeydew in the snow
chills the winter heat

Grown in the heart of winter
with the promise of summer

A block of your sugar
is all I've ever seen
Do you even live?

Dong Kui Zi

Indian Mallow Seed

Semen Abutii (sometimes Semen Malvae)

Sweet, Cold
BL, LI, SI

- ~ Promotes and unblocks
- ~ Benefits the breasts and increases lactation
- ~ Moisten the intestines and unblocks the bowels.

Door to door magpie
selling nothing but futures
and future futures

Campaigners make promises
hoping crops grow in the shade

from a frozen stream
we put our hands on the ice
and beg for water

Fu Ling

Tuckahoe, Hoelen
茯苓 (bukuryo)
Sclerotum Poriae Cocos

Sweet, Bland, Neutral
HRT, KI, LU, SP

~   Promotes urination and drains dampness
~   Strengthens the spleen and harmonizes the middle Jiao
~   Quiets the heart and calms the spirit

When the stomach screams
the whole house is awaken
and no one can dream

Hunger driving children
to wear pants and moustaches

The world could be fed
if Tuckahoe could be grown
upon rotten hearts

Guang Fang Zi

Stephania Fangchi Root
Radix Aristolochiae Fangii

Bitter, Spicy, Cold, Toxic
BL, LU

~ Sharply expels wind damp heat
~ Promotes urination and reduces edema

Bitter general
against the wind, he's standing
Plate armor crackling

In the broad field of August
1,000 wind chimes standing

Guang Fang Zi:
A charm against ill fortune
and crawling serpent

Han Fang Zi

Four Stamen Stephania Root
Radix Stephaniae Tetradrae

Bitter, Spicy, Cold, Toxic
BL, KI, SP

~ Expels wind damp and relieves pain
~ Promotes urination and reduces edema

Open the four gates
and drive out the enemy
along with your friends

At the tip of a barrel
there is no room to explain

with infrared eyes
friends often look like a foe
rarely the reverse

Hua Shi

Talc

滑石 (Kasseki)

Talcum

Sweet, Bland, Cold

BL, ST

~ Promotes urination, drains heat from the bladder
~ Clears summer heat and damp heat
~ Absorbs dampness, clears heat, and stops bleeding topically

---

Watching elephants
toss dirt and mud on their backs
summer at the zoo

my head suddenly feels warm
I powder myself with talc

in our DNA
we share as many secrets
as there are dust motes

Jin Qian Cao

Asian Moneywort, Loose Strife Herb
Herba Lysimachiae

Sweet, Salty, Bland, Slightly Cold
BL, GB, KI, LIV

~ Promotes urination and expels stoned
~ Clears damp heat in the liver and gallbladder and expels gallstones
~ Reduces toxicity and swelling

King Lysimachus
offered madness a flower
and was given the same

A mad cow rendered inert
in the presence of petals

to the ox I ask;
is it the palmates of green,
or the palm serene

Mu Tong

Armand Clematis Stem, Chocolate Vine Stem

木通 (mokutsu)

Caulis Akebiae

Bitter, Slightly Cold
BL, HRT, SI

~ Promotes urination and unblocks painful urinary dysfunction
~ Drains heat from the heart through the small intestine
~ Promotes lactation and unblocks the blood vessels

The ivory coast
sends gifts to my beloved
in bars and kisses

Some say it begins with a "k"
but a kiss starts with a "c"

If ever there proof
of a benevolent god,
one looks to Hershey's

Qu Mai

Rainbow Pink, Proud Pink Herb
Herba Dianthi

Bitter, Cold
BL, HRT, SI

~ Clears damp heat, promotes urination, and unblocks painful
   urination
~ Breaks up blood stasis and invigorates blood circulation
~ Clears heart and small intestine fire
~ Unblocks the bowels

A water busker
dancing in the flower pot
Proud pink, sweet William

Dew lining A begging bowl
cools my stomach and my heart

The 5-petal skirts
in the sun, like bubblegum
Pink upon the pink

Shi Wei

Felt Fern Leaf
Folium Pyrrosiae

Bitter, Sweet, Slightly Cold
BL, LU

~ Promotes urination and drains damp-heat from the bladder
~ Clears heat and stops bleeding
~ Clears the lungs, expels phlegm, and relieves cough

Tripping over vines
I make a bed of the dirt
a blanket of ferns

my head smashes a bad stool
forest scent cushions my fall

Check, nothing broken
I wipe a drop of white blood
a surprised bird flies

Tong Cao

Rice Paper Plant Pith
Medulla Tetrapanacis

Sweet, Bland, Slightly Cold
Lu, ST

~   Promotes urination, resolves dampness, and clears heat
~   Promotes lactation

I'll write all my ills
and deliver them to god
on rice paper Pith

of the doctor's prescription
I make a pulpy beverage

the calligrapher
writes the character "genki"
on Tong Cao circles

Yi Yi Ren

Job's Tears, Coix Seed

薏苡仁 (yokuinin)

Semen Coicis

Sweet, Bland, Slightly Cold
KI, LU, SP

~ Expels wind damp and relieves pain
~ Strengthens the spleen and resolves dampness.
~ Clears heat and expels pus
~ Clears damp heat

Unwilling actor
Job upon the stage of life
no more re-runs, please

if all the world's a stage
then where's the actors union?

They, who cast our parts
already know our Talent
and ask only for Action

Yin Chen Hao

Oriental Wormwood

茵陳蒿 (inchinko)

Herba Artemisiae Scopariae

Bitter, Slightly Cold
GB, LIV, SP, ST

~ Clears damp heat from the liver and gallbladder and relieves jaundice.
~ Clears damp heat and releases dampness

Lonesome actor drinks
enough to see the stars
that he longs to be

No one makes a manager
from green fairy's agency

Poured strait from those eyes
Her intoxicating gaze
fills his empty heart

Yu Mi Xu

Cornsilk
Stigma Maydis

Sweet, Bland, Neutral
BL, GB, LIV

~ Promotes urination, reduces edema, unblocks urinary dysfunction
~ Regulates the gallbladder and clears damp heat
~ Removes jaundice and treats wasting and thirsting disorder

Discarded clothing
From these strands, she made a doll
Dust bowl companion

Husking the corn, it feels like
how husking the corn feels like

Tempered by the sun
Her temper never showing
to her spoiled son

Ze Xie

Water Plantain Rhizome
沢瀉 (takusha)
Rhizoma Alismatis

Sweet, Bland, Cold
BL, KI

~ Promotes urination and drains dampness
~ Drains deficient kidney fire
~ Drains damp heat in the lower Jiao and settles Ministerial fire

---

Dog leaps from a truck
and pisses on a flower
hops back in the cab

both seem perfectly happy
to be part of this tableau

The flowers don't care
if nourishment is yellow
or if it is clear

Zhu Ling

Griffolia, Umbel Polypore Mushroom

猪苓 (Chorei)

Sclerotum Polyporus

Sweet, Bland, Slightly Cool
KI, SP, BL

~ Promotes urination and drains dampness
~ Dispels damp heat with turbid dysfunction

A wise man once said
a parasol is to rain
as sun is to moon

From beneath the umbrella
the whole world looks soggy

The weight of raindrops
isn't counted in ounces
nor measured in grams

Herbs That Drain Downward

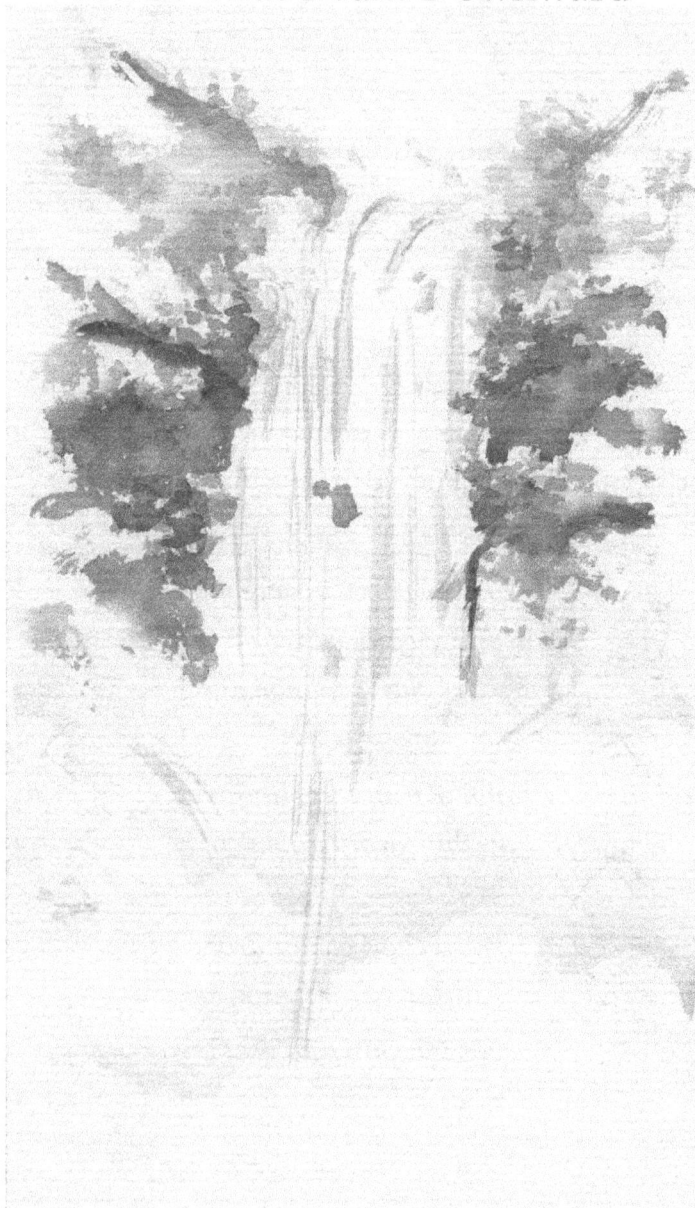

Ba Dou

Croton Seed

巴豆 (Hazu)

Fructud Crotonis

Spicy, Hot, Toxic
LI, LU, ST

~ Vigorously purges and warmly unblocks
~ Drives out water and reduces edema
~ Dissolves clogged phlegm and improves the condition of the throat
~ Promotes healing of abscesses and ulcers topically

No one will answer
no matter how loud you knock
Oh, battering ram

Whatever you are selling
I am not interested

Selling liberty?
Your pitch could use improvement
and my door needs fixed

Da Huang

Rhubarb Root and Rhizome

大黄 (daio)

Radix et Rhizoma Rhei

Bitter, Cold
HRT, LI, LIV, ST

~ Drains heat and purges accumulations
~ Drains heat from the blood
~ Clears heat and fire, transforms dampness, and promotes urination
~ Invigorates the blood and dispels blood stasis
~ Clears heat and reduces fire toxicity

Corruptions limit;
We accept bitter and cold
to fight the putrid

Now the battle is over
and we feel fully drained

For 17 days
the Great Yellow is in charge
We live as Spartans

Fan Xie Ye

Senna Leaf
Folium Sennae

Sweet, Bitter, Cold
LI

~ Drains downward, guides out stagnation
~ Eliminates excess heat and summer heat

Da Huang's junior;
he takes knives and hands out forks
turns stink into sweet

if you beat a mule to death
it cannot take you forward

Traffic at a halt
A man curses his cabbie
Summer in New York

Gan Sui

Euphorbie Root
Radix Kansui

Bitter, Sweet, Cold, Toxic
KI, LI, LU

~ Drains water downward and drives out congested fluid
~ Expels Phlegm
~ Clears heat, reduces swellings, and softens hardenings

There was two lines
one of them was given pink
There were two lines

Is it death or the farmer
who winnows wheat from the chaff

5 stages of grief
Starts with cleaning out your desk
ends in classifieds

Huo Ma Ren

Hemp Seed
Semen Cannabis

Sweet, Neutral
LI, SP, ST

~ Lubricates, and nourishes the intestines and hair
~ Mildly nourishes Yin, clears heat, and promotes the healing of
  sores

She is watching me
as I fill the cup half way
discarding the rest

beheld by her eyes and hand
the taboo becomes product

A weekend of joy.
Has the memory faded
from my bladder?

Lu Hui

Dried Aloe Juice Concentrate
Aloe

Bitter, Cold
LI, LIV, ST

~ Drains fire and guides out accumulation
~ Kills parasites and strengthens stomach
~ Clears heat and cools the liver

Across the dessert
The yucca prods the workers
the aloe heals them

Spears bristling them forward
spears that prevent regression

Mother and child
wade across the shallow end
Rio Grand crossing

Mang Xiao

Mirabilite, Glauber's Salt, Sodium Sulfate
芒硝 (Bosho)
Natrii Sulfas

Bitter, Salty, Spicy, Very Cold
LI, ST

~ Purges accumulations, guides out stagnation, soften hardness, and moistens dryness
~ Clears heat, drains fire, and reduces swelling

After the monsoon
the photo albums floating
across the basement

will you make new memories
or was the past more buoyant?

Above the flotsam
the future is hard to see
through the past's jetsam

Qian Niu Zi

Morning Glory Seeds
Semen Pharbitidis

Bitter, Spicy, Cold, Slightly Toxic
KI, LI, LU, SI

~ Drives out water through urine and stool
~ Descends lung Qi and drives out phlegm and mucus
~ Unblocks the bowels and removes damp heat
~ Expels intestinal parasites and reduces food stagnation

The sun has risen
counting morning glory seeds
sun rises again

who hid syllables of god
in such a minuscule pods?

The holy verse read
"not the human consumption"
prayer envelopes

Shang Lu

Poke Root
Radix Phytolaccae

Bitter, Cold, Toxic
BL, KI, LI, SP

~ Drives out water through the stool and urine
~ Reduces sores and carbuncles topically
~ Removes phlegm, stops cough, and resolves lumps
~ Reduces swelling and nodules

At the speed limit
or several miles over
the fare is the same

I get one word in English
to the thousand in his phone

To the yellow thunderbolt
there is no pain or trouble
not solved with a tip

Yu Li Ren

Bush Cherry Pit
Semen Pruni

Bitter, Spicy, Sweet, Neutral
LI, SI, SP

~   Moistens intestines and unblocks the bowel
~   Promotes urination and reduces edema in the legs.

Growing by gravel
Crimped green leaf, red berry
Backyard bush berry

In summer, Gian and I
turn the red shrub green

We once dug a hole
for no other reason
than to dig a whole

Yuan Hua

Lilac Daphne Flower
Flos Genkwa

Bitter, Spicy, Warm, Toxic
KI, LI, LU

~ Drains water downward, drives out congested fluid, and promotes urination
~ Resolves phlegm and stops cough
~ Kills parasites topically

Inhaling vapors
he sees my engine failing
Oil shop oracle

My tribute displeases him
20% off coupon

The black ritual;
The impure is driven out
golden crude poured in

Herbs That Drain Fire

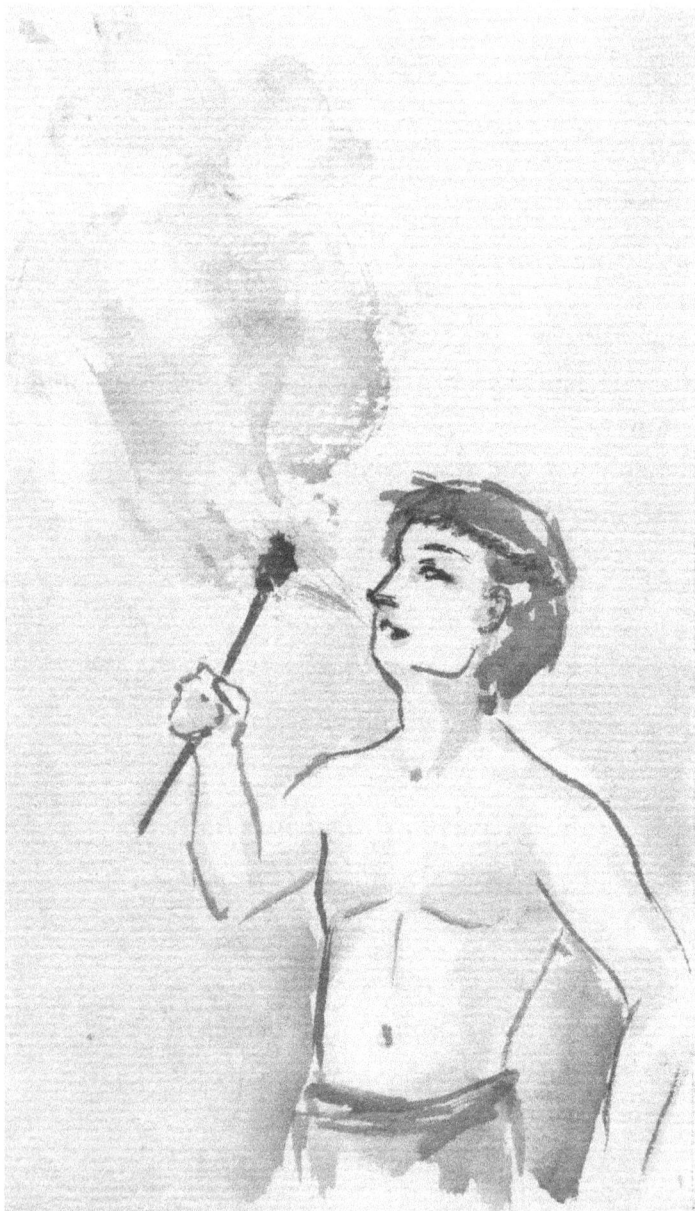

Dan Zhu Ye

Bamboo leaves and Stem
淡竹葉 (takuchikuyo)
Herba Lophatheri

Sweet, Bland, Cold
HRT, SI, ST

~ Clears heat with irritability and thirst
~ Promotes urination and clears damp heat

Cellulose hoarder
the panda consumes his weight
in tubes of grasses

Everyone loves a panda
yet forget it is a bear

In misty china
Rangers toil to preserve
an ink brush paining

Gu Jing Cao

Buerger Pipewort Flower
Flos Eriocauli

Sweet, Neutral
LIV, ST

~   Disperse wind heat in the liver channel and brightens the eyes

---

For months in japan
I wondered who played two notes
walking down the street

I mistook the produce call
for someone on recorder

pi .... Pipaaaaa
the vegetable ambulance
driving down my block

Han Shui Shi

Red Gypsum, Calcite
Glauberitum

Salty, Spicy, Cold
HRT, KI, ST

~ Expels summer heat
~ Clears heat and drains fire
~ Burns and sores topically
~ Promotes urination and reduces edema
~ Directs fire downward and softens hardness

On the cul-de-sac
she raises her crystal wand
made of acrylic

surely its mythic amber
and not a plastic resin

in those hands of hers
that can barely hold the world
cheap becomes precious

Jue Ming Zi / Cao Jue Ming

Fetid Cassia Seed, Sickle Senna Seed
決明子 (ketsumeishi)
Semen Cassiae

Bitter, Salty, Sweet, Slightly Cold
KI, LI, LIV

~ Clears the vision and expels wind heat
~ Calms the liver and anchors liver Yang
~ Moistens intestines and unblocks the bowels
~ Lowers blood pressure and serum cholesterol

Pungent on pungent
the seeds of sickle senna
perfume my spice rack

Walking into my kitchen
every smell a tale

A biography
told in stains and memories
of every meal cooked

Lian Zi Xin

Lotus Plumule
Plumula Nelumbinis

Bitter, Cold
HRT, PC

~ Drains heart fire and relieves irritability
~ Stops bleeding and binds the essence

Heart inside the heart
the yellow inside the pink
lightning in the night

In the flower's purity
Pandora left her free will

Plucking the plummule
The flower still calls for bees
produces no seed

Lu Gen

Reed Rhizome
Rhizoma Phragmitis

Sweet, Cold
LU, ST

~ Clears heat and irritation from the lungs and stomach
~ Clears stomach heat and regulates stomach Qi
~ Clears heat and promotes urination
~ Relieves vomiting and belching
~ Encourages rashes to surface
~ Eases food poisoning

The dirt of the week
is placed on a tiny hook
and cast to the fish

The gum from the park permits
drawing bars on the windshield

Coke over Pepsi
and earthworms over leaches
every Saturday

Mi Meng Hua

Pale Butterfly Bush Flower
Flos Buddlejae

Sweet, Slightly Cool
LIV

~   Benefits the eyes and clears the liver
~   Moistens liver dryness

Perfect handwriting
A voice as loud as silence
Shy English student

Emphasizing in thick lines
bold, and underlined twice

I only got "mmm"
when enlightenment was found
Never "wakata"

Qing Xiang Zi

Silver Quail-Grass Seed
Semen Celosiae

Sweet, Slightly Cool
LIV

~ Strongly drains liver fire and clears wind heat
~ Treats hypertension due to liver yang rising
~ Improves vision

Lost in Hakone
soft music pumped into fog
a quail, running

I would call it "Brigadoon"
and everyone understood

It was my first time
and every time I return
a new Babylon

Shi Gao

Gypsum

石膏 (Sekko)

Gypsum Fibrosum

Spicy, Sweet, Very Cold
LU, ST

~ The most important herb to clear internal heat, especially in the qi and yang ming levels.
~ Clears excess lung heat
~ Clears blazing stomach fire
~ Topically for eczema, burns, ulcerated sores, and wounds

A dose of gypsum
Magma becomes an island
the world starts to cool

the deep cold of the ocean
crashing against fresh basalt

We start to warm up
when we stop resisting it
Pacific Ocean

Xia Ku Cao

Selfheal Spike
夏枯草 (Kagoso)
Spica Prunellae

Bitter, Spicy, Cold
GB, LIV

~ Clears liver fire and brightens the eyes
~ Clears heat and dissipates nodules
~ Treats hypertension accompanied by liver fire or yang rising.

It does not bandage
It only stops the burning
in a scorched heart

medicine kit in my chest
the key, deep in my liver

A cut in her heart
She matches it on her arm
just to watch it heal

Xiong Dan

Bear Gallbladder

Vessica Fella Ursi

Bitter, Cold
GB, HRT, LIV, SP

~   Clears heat from the heart and liver and alleviates spasms
~   Clears and drains liver heat and benefits the eyes
~   Topically to relieve fire toxicity

Crated wilderness
isn't a substitute for
the bite of nature

Plastic piping does not give
what the wild wood crafted

tapping suffering
without the taste of courage
is dry and useless

Ye Ming Sha

Bat Guano

Faeces Vespertilionis

Spicy, Cold
LIV

~ Clears liver and improves vision and improves night blindness
~ Disperses blood stasis and bruising

Shining night stand
gives a 2nd chance
to flying rat shit

what is good for the flower
might not be good for the mouth

A gift mined from caves
only the saints could find it
A gift mind from caves

Zhi Mu

Know Mother Root
知母 (chimo)
Rhizoma Anemarrhenae

Bitter, Sweet, Cold
KI, LU, ST

~ Clears heat and drains fire from the lung and stomach
~ Nourishes Yin and moistens dryness
~ Generates fluids and clears deficient fire
~ Ameliorates the dryness of tonifying and warming herbs

Who would take value
in doctors and literature
when mother knows best

Chicken soup can cure the plague
grilled cheese reverses the flu

There's none who question
what faith lies between magic
and the word of mom

Zhi Zi

Cape Jasmine Fruit
Fructus Gardeniae

Bitter, Cold
HRT, LIV, LU, ST, TB

~ Clears heat, fire, and reduces irritability
~ Drains damp heat in the lower Jiao and triple burner
~ Cools the blood, stops bleeding, and relieves toxicity
~ Topically for swelling.

The fisherman's wife
blowing kisses to the waves
Seaside jasmine bush

White capped waves reaching up
white capped flowers reaching down

the scent of blossoms
and the spray of the ocean
perfume of Venus

Herbs That Expel Parasites

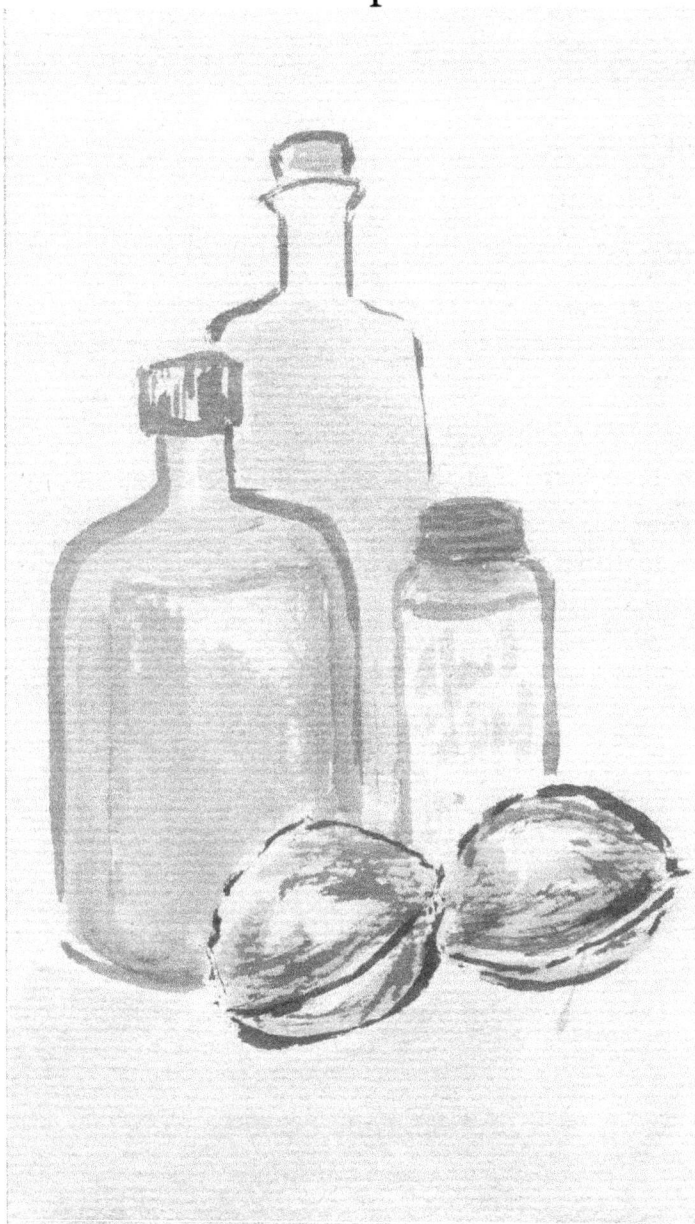

Bing Lang

Betel Nut

檳榔子 (Binrojin)

Semen Arecae

Acrid, Bitter, Warm
LI, ST

~ Kills parasites, especially tapeworms
~ Promote movement of Qi, reduce stagnation, drains down and unblocks the bowels
~ Promote urination and relieves nausea
~ Treats malarial disorder

Cherry blossom stains
on the curry shop sidewalk
Betel nut petals

In the North, a drink that kills
In the South, a chew that lives

White nut turning red
draining and expelling
the heats of India

Chang Shan

Feverflower Root
Rhizoma Dichroae

Bitter, Spicy, Cold, Toxic
HRT, LIV, LU

~ Checks malarial conditions and kills parasites
~ Induces vomiting to expel phlegm in the chest

Customer and clerk
argue over 12 cents
Bitter fights bitter

The rest of the line reflects
on what is good behavior

The next in the line
gives both of them a quarter
buying sheepish looks

Guan Zhong

Shield Fern
Rhizoma Dryopteris

Bitter, Cold, Slightly Toxic
LIV, ST

~ Kills parasites
~ Drains heat and relieves fire toxicity
~ Cools the blood and stops bleeding

A stick for a sword
a kitten for a dragon
a fern for a shield

the cat goes skittering off
I thank the knight for his help

His trusty wizard
I slay monsters with day-glo
and a plug-in light

Nan Gua Zi

Red Squash Seed
Semen Cucurbitae Moschatae

Sweet, Neutral
LI, ST

~ Expels parasites and alleviates pain
~ Benefits post-partum fluid movement

I carved out his head
threw away his brain matter
and roasted his dreams

My trophy on the front porch
a symbol of victory

Before all is lost
I grant him enlightenment
Jack-o-Lantern

Herbs That Extinguish Wind and Tremors

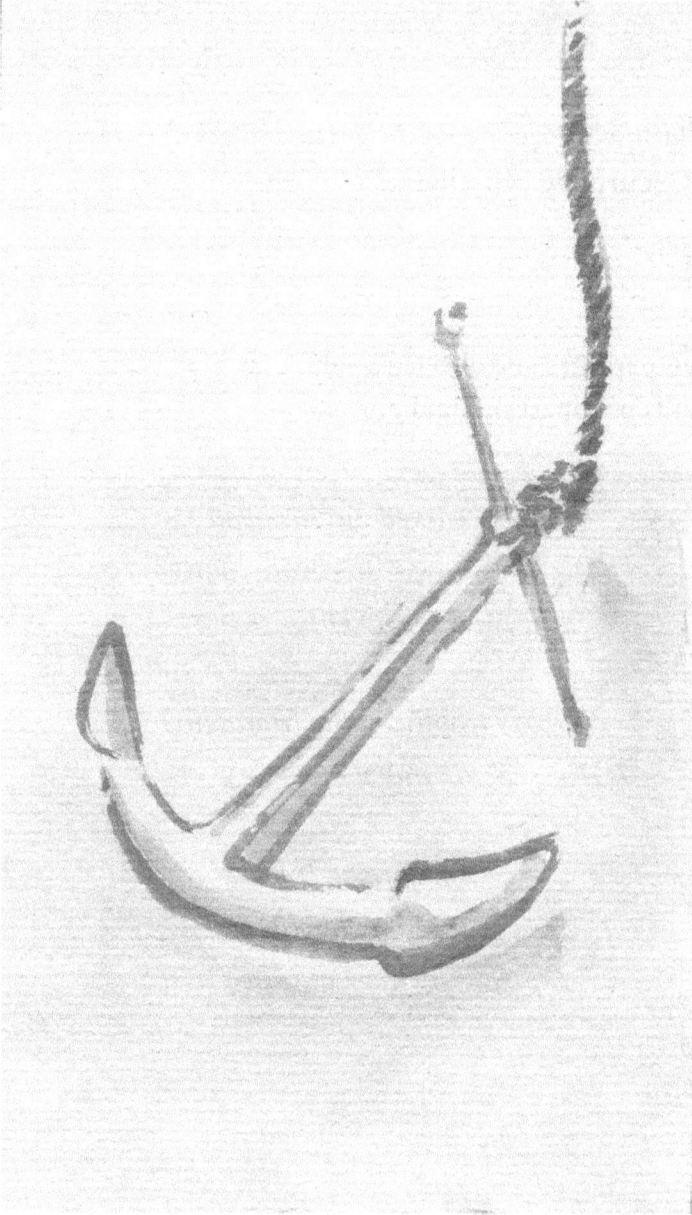

Bai Ji Li / Ci Ji Li

Caltrop Fruit

蒺藜子 (刺蒺藜) (Shitsurishi)

Fructus Tribuli

Bitter, Spicy, Neutral
LIV

~ Calms the liver and anchors the yang
~ Dredges liver Qi, extinguishes liver fire, and disperses stagnation and clumping
~ Treats liver Yang rising with headaches and eye irritation
~ Expels wind and stops itching.

Late in the summer
I curse the fruits of the sun
and grab my bare foot

The sting of injustice
outlasts the sting of the seed

I crush the caltrops
A tea that stings my stressors
and defends my heart

Di Long

Minor Blue-Green Earth Dragon, Earthworm
Lumbricus

Salty, Cold
BL, LIV, LU, SP

~ Drains liver heat, extinguishes wind, and stops spasms and convulsions
~ Clears lung heat and calms wheezing.
~ Clears heat in the channels and promotes movement
~ Clears heat and promotes urination
~ Treats blood pressure associated with liver yang rising.

In the rain, come up
and dance along the sidewalk
until the sky clears

Minor blue-green earth dragon
is what medics call the worm

Who could feel disgust
for the one who bites the hook
and ploughs the garden

Gou Teng

Uncaria Vine, Gambir, Cat's Claw

釣藤鈎 (Chotoko)

Ramulus cum Uncis Uncariae

Sweet, Slightly Cold
LIV, PC

~ Extinguishes wind and alleviates spasms
~ Drains liver heat and pacifies liver Yang
~ Releases the exterior, especially in tension headaches

Calling me hither
with the same hand it uses
to drive me away

Who would make such a creature
who shows love with a razor?

Soft, and then sharpness
longing turning to fury
cats furry belly

Ling Yang Jiao

Antelope Horn
羚羊角 (Reiyokaku)
Cornu Antelopis

Salty, Cold
HRT, LIV

~ Extinguishes wind, controls spasms, and drains liver heat
~ Calms the liver, improves vision, and anchors the yang
~ Drains heat and fire toxicity

Fence on the prairie
holding back the coyote
over slips two prongs

For a moment, suspended
life and death over pickets

A dash and a leap
A mother returning home
A meal escapes

Quan Xie

Scorpion
Buthus Martensi

Salty, Spicy, Neutral, Toxic
LIV

~ Extinguishes liver wind and strongly stops tremors
~ Strongly clears fire toxins and nodules
~ Unblocks the collaterals, tracks down wind, and stops pain

Above Mt. Casper
underneath the oil shale
fossils and cousins

Test you bravery at night
and watch them glow like plastic

They fluoresce no more
Mixing them in paper bags
for tremmoring patients

Shi Jue Ming

Abalone Shell

Concha Haliotidis

Salty, Cold
KI, LIV

~ Drains liver fire, descends and anchors rising yang, and pacifies the lover
~ Improves the vision and clears visual obstructions
~ Calms internal wind, clears stomach fire and stops pain

On our honeymoon
we try the conch at dinner
because we are in love

It is the first of many
experiments we will share

Some left on the plate
Neither of us like the taste
but we love the flavor

Tian Ma

Heavenly Hemp Rhizome
Rhizoma Gastrodiae

Sweet, Neutral
LIV

~ Calms the liver, extinguishes liver wind from either heat or cold
  patterns, and stops spasms and tremors
~ Extinguishes wind, alleviates pain, and subdues rising liver Yang
~ Disperse painful obstruction due to wind phlegm

Nothing narcotic
in this vinegared tuber
Nothing except peace

Taste like stale potato chips
Looks and smells about the same

Some things in poor taste,
like bad jokes and bland herbs,
hide wisdom and peace

Wu Gong

Centipede
Scolopendra

Spicy, Warm, Toxic
LIV

~ Extinguishes wind and stops spasms
~ Dissipates toxins and nodules and relieves fire toxins
~ Unblocks the collaterals and stops pain

A stick through the head
they latch on and attack it
Violent medicine

Attacking all during life
Attacking wind after death

Shaking out my boots
to the tatami it drops
Shaking in my boots

Herbs That Invigorate Blood

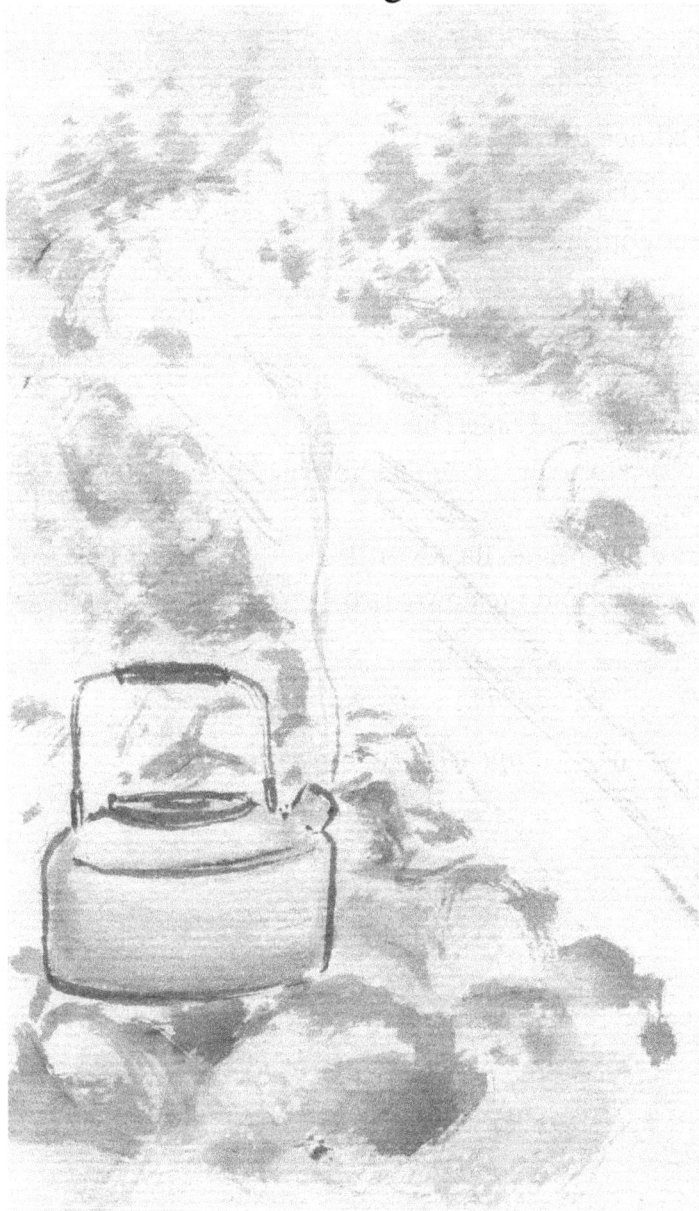

Huai Niu Xi

White Oxknee Root
牛膝 (Goshitsu)
Radix Achyranthis Bidentatae

Bitter, Sour, Neutral
KI, LIV

~ Invigorates blood expels blood stasis
~ Nourishes liver and kidney Yin, strengthens the sinews, bones, and joints
~ Clears damp heat in the lower Jiao
~ Brings blood and fire downward

The sedge-hat farmers
compelled to walk behind them
as they till the field

The oxen pull the farmer
The farmer pushes the ox

No energy lost
when pushing comes from pulling
and pull comes to push

Chi Shao

Red Peony Root
Radix Paeoniae Rubra

Bitter, Sour, Slightly Cold
LIV, SP

~ Invigorates blood and dispels stasis
~ Clears heat and cools the blood
~ Clears liver fire and relieves eye pain

The scent of coyness
Peony with blood for sap
blushes at my touch

My heart runs flush with vigor
when your pollen is let loose

Plucking at your dress
your evergreen modesty
tastes good in my cup

Chuan Shan Jia

Pangolin Anteater scales
Squama Manitis

Salty, Cool
LIV, ST

~ Disperses blood stasis, unblocks menses, and promotes lactation
~ Reduces swellings and promotes discharge of pus
~ Expels wind damp from the channels.

In search of scales
who would disassemble
god's artwork

He gives away a bouquet
and someone steals a vase

At a certain point
scarcity becomes prayer

Chuan Xiong

Szechwan Lovage Rhizome

川芎 (Senkyo)

Rhizoma Chuanxiong

Spicy, Warm
GB, LIV, PC

~ Invigorate blood, promote movement of Qi
~ Expels wind and alleviates pain
~ Clears headache pain and tension

I have a craving
sticky sour and saccharine
Lovage and gummies

The flavors of adulthood
can't match the taste of youth

No one can eat it
and appear adult
Slice of watermelon

Dan Shen

Red Sage Root
Radix Salviae Miltiorrhizae

Bitter, Slightly Cold
HRT, LIV, PC

~ Invigorate blood and breaks up blood stasis in lower abdomen
~ Clear heat and soothe irritability
~ Cools the blood and reduces abscesses
~ Nourishes the blood and calms the spirit

Truth burns, like a brand
We reach out our arms and wince
holding hot iron

they tell us that we can't hold
and that we cannot release

A heard of mad monks
pastoral and violent
stampede in my mind

E Zhu

Zedoary Root
Rhizoma Curcumae Zedoariae

Bitter, Spicy, Warm
LIV, SP

~ Invigorates the blood, promotes the movement of Qi, alleviates
  pain
~ Dissolve accumulations, stagnation, and pain

When you were sick
I walked a million miles
to hide my weakness

I would call you on the phone
and pray to hear your voicemail

I grew so small
hoping the patent bottle
could keep me hidden

Hong Hua

Safflower
紅花 (Koka)
Flos Carthami

Spicy, Warm
HRT, LIV

~ Invigorates the blood and unblocks menstruation
~ Dispels blood stasis and alleviates pain

Deep in the fire
the meat begins to sizzle
fat dribbles on coals

Sticks, filthy moments ago
now serve as our chopsticks

Before they can burst
we spear the german sausage
with a pocket knife

Hu Zhang

Japanese Knotweed Rhizome
Rhizoma Poligoni Cuspidati

Bitter, Cold
GB, LIV, LU

~ Invigorates blood, dispels stasis, and unblocks the channels
~ Clears heat and resolves dampness
~ Drains heat and transforms phlegm
~ Discharges toxins and disperses swelling

The loom and shuttle
in my grandparent's basements
I imagine the sound

Playing string and percussion
a single tune lasting weeks

My scratchy blanket
has grown much softer
since my grandma died

Ji Xue Teng

Millettia Root and Vine
Caulis Spatholobi

Bitter, Sweet, Warm
HRI, LIV, SP

~ Invigorates the movement of blood and tonifies the blood
~ Invigorate the channels and relax the sinews

Three flavors today
if you were to consume me;
bitter, sweet, and warm

In my backyard, a garden
weeds and petunias complete

Wild tomatoes
plentiful and delicious
making my mouth itch

Jiang Huang

Tumeric

Rhizoma Curcumae Longae

Bitter, Spicy, Warm
LIV, SP, ST

~ Invigorate the blood, eliminates blood stasis, and unblock menses
~ Promote the movement of Qi and opens the channels
~ Expels wind, invigorates the blood, and reduces swelling

Different qualities
yet seen through the same eyes
Printed photographs

no one takes pictures to show
they take them to remember

"you should have been there
hooded field, sunset water"
-dry ginger

Lu Lu Tong

Liquidamber, Sweetgum Fruit
Fructus Liquidamberis

Bitter, Neutral
LIV, ST

~ Promotes movement of qi and invigorates the blood, opens middle
  Jiao, and unblocks the channels
~ Promotes urination and expels wind
~ Promotes lactation
~ Treats allergies

Cleaning up my lawn
the next platonic solid
is the sweetgum shell

caught using Menger's sponge
to clean up my messy meth

Sum of existence:
No volume, endless surface
and gum tree seedpods

Mo Yao

Myrrh
Resina Commiphorae

Bitter, Neutral
HRT, LIV, SP

~ Invigorate blood, dispel blood stasis, reduces swelling and alleviate pain
~ Promotes healing and generates flesh

They gave him myrrh
because no life is lived
without hurt and healing

There are no bands of gold
that can brace a bleeding heart

Even the divine
loose a tusk or an eye,
or take with them scars

Ru Xiang

Boswellia, Frankincense
Gummi Olibani

Bitter, Spicy, Warm
HRT, LIV, SP

~ Invigorates blood and increases the movement of Qi
~ Relax the sinews, invigorates the channels, and alleviates pain
~ Reduces swellings and generates flesh

In the Sahara
you ask a tree to cry
to avoid weeping

Who is to say it is sad?
It could be weeping with joy

A blood donation
irrregardless of species
or even phylum

San Leng

Burr-Reed Rhizome

Rhizoma Sparganii

Bitter, Spicy, Neutral
LIV, SP

~ Breaks up blood stasis, promotes movement of Qi, and alleviates pain
~ Dissolves accumulations and regulates menstruation

Grit polishes rock
sandpaper polishes wood
life polishes life

diamonds colliding in space
Atoms colliding at CERN

little in nothing
chased by Shrodinger's cat
creates everything

Shui Zhi

Leech

Hirudo

Bitter, Salty, Neutral, Slightly Toxic (Toxic to pregnancy)
BL, LIV

~ Breaks up blood stasis and reduces masses
~ Clears water passages

Mud under my sock
I flick it....!
I flick flick flick it!

A lion thrashing madly
a painless thorn in his foot

He flicked his lighter
The mud became animate
and fell to the ground

Si Gua Luo

Loofah

Fructus Luffae Retinervus

Sweet, Neutral
LIV, LU, ST

~ Resolves toxicity and reduces swelling
~ Unblocks the channels and collaterals in the breast
~ Unblocks the channels and collaterals and dispels Wind
~ Expels phlegm and cough from lung heat

I scrub with a Fruit
and yet at the same time
I eat my washcloth

Can you scrub out that last poem?
Its foul taste is lingering

Triton, a practical god
who makes tool, food, and fish all one
in service of all

Su Mu

Sappan Wood
蘇木 (Soboku)
Lignum Sappan

Salty, Spicy, Sweet, Neutral
HRT, LIV, SP

~ Invigorates blood, reduces swelling, opens the channels, and
  alleviates pain
~ Stops bleeding

From my balcony
twilight cobblestone road
the clack of wood heels

a rectangle firefly
follows her into the dark

her voice now fading
I can still hear her wood soul
going down the road

Tao Ren

Peach Kernel
桃仁 (Tonin)
Semen Persicae

Bitter, Sweet, Neutral
HRT, LI, LIV, LU

~ Breaks up blood stasis and invigorates the blood
~ Moistens intestines and unblock the bowels
~ Drains abscesses

Soft, hard, then bitter
three lifetimes held in one hand
The immortal's peach

When bitter does not offend
the sweetness can be found

Unpacking the peach kernels
I hope that somebody
enjoyed the Fruit

Tu Bie Chong

Wingless Cockroach

土鳖虫 (Shachu)

Eupolyphaga / Steleophaga

Salty, Cold, Slightly Toxic
HRT, LIV, SP

~ Breaks up and drives out blood stasis, invigorates circulation, and disperses masses
~ Renews and rebuilds joints, sinews, and bones

How come our elders
who are older than mankind
do not get respect

I feel that we should honor
those who live without a head

Who'll remember us
when we chop off our own head?
None, but the cockroach

Wa Leng Zi

Ark shell, Cockle shell
Concha Arcae

Salty, Neutral
LIV, LU, SP

~ Invigorates the blood, dissolve phlegm, softens abdominal masses,
   and resolves stagnation
~ Absorb acid and alleviate pain

To the sea, a home
to the cockle, its an ark
to my foot, a pain

Salt and sand in my cut foot
I imagine I'm poisoned

On our honeymoon
we were afraid of the sea,
the benevolent sea

Wang Bu Liu Xing

Cow Soapwort Seeds
Semen Vaccariae

Bitter, Neutral
LIV, ST

~ Invigorates the blood and channels and promotes the movement of blood
~ Reducing swelling and drains abscesses
~ Promotes healing of cut wounds

A steak, milk, and cheese
I'm always asking of her
giving as if it's nothing

I saw you frolic in spring
and yet, I can still eat you

I can't not eat you
But I have not learned yet
how I say thank you

Wu Ling Zhi

Flying Squirrel Feces

Excrementum Trogopteri seu Pteromi

Bitter, Salty, Warm
LIV

~ Invigorates the blood, relieves pain, and dispels blood stasis
~ Transforms stasis, stop bleeding, and eliminates toxins

Religious trinket
made of plastic and spray paint
god still lives in there

it is not in the carving
it's in the salesman's hand

Buyer and seller
To make the magic beans grow
it takes perfect faith

Xue Jie

Sanguis Draconis, Dragon's Blood
Resina Daemonoropis

Sweet, Salty, Neutral
HRT, LIV

~ Dispels blood stasis, relieves pain, and invigorates the blood
~ Protects decay of ulcer's surface and generates flesh
~ Stops bleeding topically

Two pricks, small and big
The tube goes from clear to red
The bay fills slowly

I imagine dividends
paid against my needle pain

Everything borrowed
is shared, person to person
Eternal living

Yan Hu Suo

Corydalis Root

延胡索 (Engosaku)

Rhizoma Corydalis

Bitter, Spicy, Warm
HRT, LIV, ST

~ Invigorates blood, moves Qi, and strongly alleviates pain
~ Induces and prolongs sleep

Heroine when drunk
and a doctor when sober
Corydalis Root

He doesn't overthink it
when I take away his thoughts

Once, while on the clock
he was invited to drink
I declined-

Yi Mu Cao

Chinese Motherwort

益母草 (Yakumoso)

Herba Leonuri

Bitter, Spicy, Slightly Cold
BL, HRT, LIV

~ Invigorates the blood, dispels stasis, and regulates menses
~ Promotes urination and reduces swelling
~ Clears heat and resolves toxicity

A knight at the gate
They call him the lion heart
they call her a him

Underneath her chest armor
straps, bandages, and truth

Defend her gender
or defend her family
it was his choice to make

Yu Jin

Curcuma Tuber

鬱金 (Ukon)

Radix Curcumae

Bitter, Spicy, Cold
HRT, LIV, LU

~ Invigorates the blood, break up stasis, and helps heal chronic sores
~ Promotes movement of Qi
~ Clears heat and cools the blood
~ Benefits the gallbladder and reduces jaundice

Only "false saffron"
makes the sun rise underground
at a price for all

who can admire a king
hiding in a palanquin?

The yellow of piss
is the same as brass and gold
which one do you wear?

Yue Ji Hua

China Tea Rose, Moon-season Rose
Flos Rosae Chinensis

Sweet, Warm
LIV

~   Invigorates blood and regulates menses
~   Reduces swelling and regulates Qi

The streetlight goes out
we find our way to the roses
by Luna's lantern

Pink roses blushing to red
the smell of crushed grass

How I long to go back
but I could never go back
even if I was there

Ze Lan

Bugleweed
Herba Lycopi

Bitter, Spicy, Slightly Warm
LIV, SP

~ Promotes the movement of blood, dispels stasis and promotes menstruation
~ Promotes urination and disperses swelling

This morning I dreamed
ocean views on mountain tops
the smell of warm rugs

Sitting in the bungalow
sunlight and the smell of wood

I never want to leave
Bugs and spiders deter me
from returning home

Zi Ran Tong

Pyrite

Pyritum

Spicy, Neutral
LIV

~ Dispels blood stasis, relieves pain, and promotes healing of bones
   and sinews

Iron or arum
when I see it on my hand
it is worth the same

Appraiser looks at my ring
I once felt so ashamed

A modern artifact
it is not the first lifetime
I have worn this ring

Herbs That Nourish the Heart and Calm the Spirit

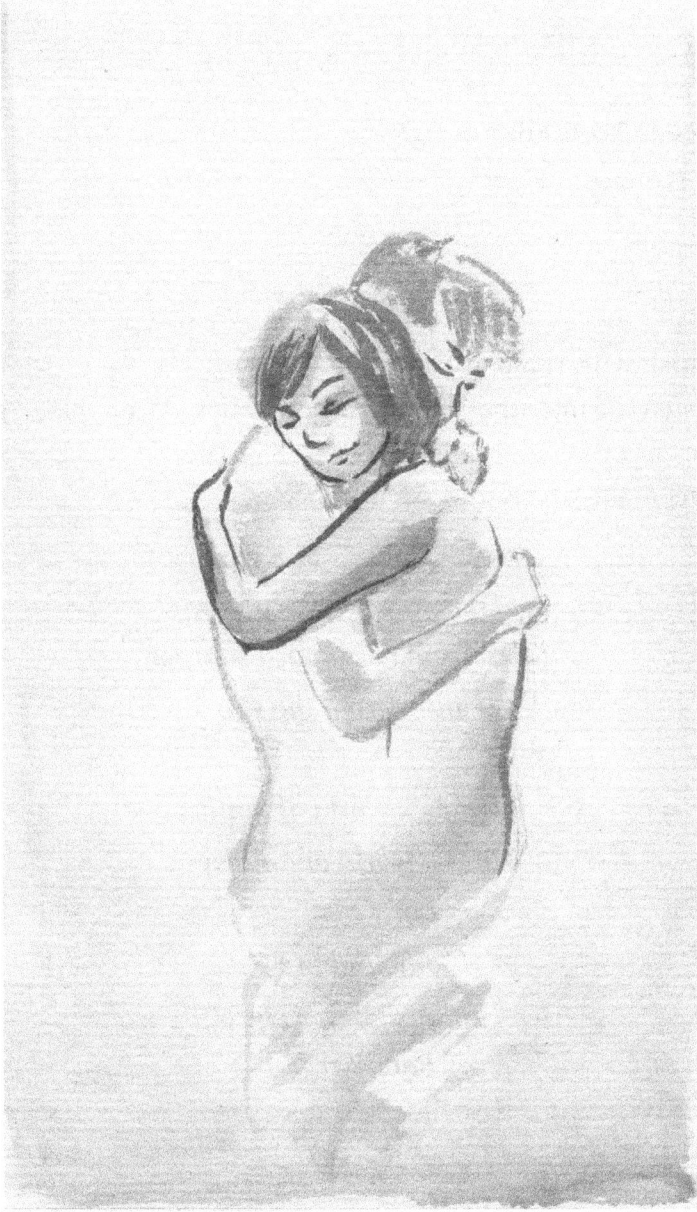

Bai Zi Ren

Biota Seed, Arborvitae Seed
Semen Thujae

Sweet, Neutral
HRT, KI, LI

~ Nourishes heart blood, calms the spirit
~ Moisten the intestines and unblocks the bowel from blood and Yin deficiency
~ Clears night-sweats due to Yin deficiency

Tree shades my window
My screen looks much sharper
hiding from the sun

I escape a world of fantasy
into a world of fantasy

I sometimes regret
I almost never regret
I don't regret

He Huan Pi

Silktree, Mimosa Tree, Albizzia Bark
Cortex Albiziae

Sweet, Neutral
HRT, LIV, LU

~ Calms the spirit and relieves constrained emotions
~ Focuses the mind and draws in happiness
~ Invigorates the blood, alleviates pain, and joins the sinews and bones
~ Regulates Qi, relieves pain, dissipates swelling and abscesses

---

My favorite herb
does exactly what it's told
gathering happiness

He Huan Hua and He Huan Pi
"Panax Emotionalis"

can no one find you?
I rarely saw your name
being called for

Suan Zao Ren

Spiny Zizyphus, Sour Jujube Seed
酸棗仁 (Sansonin)
Semen Zizyphi Spinosae

Sweet, Sour, Neutral
GB, HRT, LIV, SP

~   Nourishes the heart Yin, tonifies liver blood, quiets the spirit
~   Prevents spontaneous sweating and night-sweats.

A stuffed big horn
no bigger than a kitten
guards me from the night

of all my stuffed animals
he never stopped being real

Now he watches me
as he has always watched me
from the top of my book stack

Ye Jiao Teng

Fleeceflower caulis
Caulis Polygoni Multiflori

Sweet, Slightly Bitter, Neutral
HRT, LIV

~ Calms the spirit and nourishes the heart Yin and blood
~ Unblocks the channels and disperses wind damp
~ Alleviates itching and astringes sweat

Only my body
with no regard for my heart
outgrew my sweater

Every loop and hook for me
About 6 sizes to small

Found a solution
to the heartbreak of growing
Now, I ask for scarves

Yuan Zhi

Chinese Senega, Thin-Leaf Milkwort Root
遠志 (Onji)
Radix Polygalae

Acrid, Spicy, Slightly Warm
HRT, LU

~ Calms the spirit, quiets the heart, and clears the path between the kidney and heart
~ Expels phlegm from the lungs, clears the orifices, and stops cough
~ Reduces abscesses and dissipate swellings

Wrapped in a blanket
lullaby and croopy cough
Held, eyes to the stars

Everything big was so small
Everything small was so big

Deep in a fever
I made it to the front door
before someone stopped me

Herbs That Open Orifices

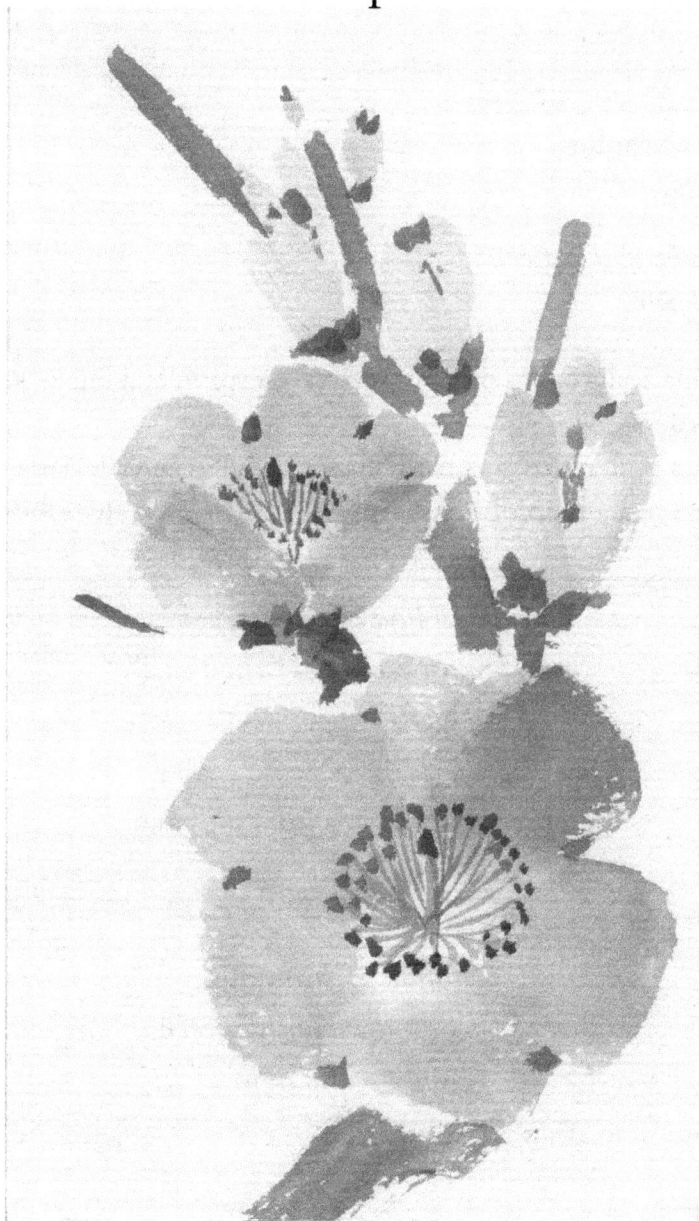

Bing Pian

Borneo Camphor
Borneolum

Acrid, Bitter, Slightly Cool,
HRT, LU, SP

~ Aromatically opens orifices, revives the spirit, and unblocks closed
  disorders
~ Clears heat, relieves pain, dissipates nodules, and alleviates itching
~ Clears heat, drains fire, resolves toxicity, and brightens the eyes

---

I had a friend
who almost renamed "The Pearl"
as "The Peppermint"

He took the forage from the cows
and fed it to aristocrats

A man of the mint
who was known for his green
I sip on him now

Niu Huang

Cattle Bezoar
牛黄 (Goo)
Calculus Bovis

Bitter, Cool
HRT, LIV

~ Clears the heart, opens the orifices, awakens the spirit, and
  vaporizes phlegm
~ Clears the liver, relieves toxicity, extinguishes wind, and stops
  tremors
~ Drains heat and relieves fire toxicity

Mistaken relief
The burden of bezoar
is best when removed

They are smarter than we think
We would paint their fences white

Manager's burden
made easier by the staff
they took on the Ark

She Xiang

Deer Musk

麝香 (Jako)

Secretio Mochus

Spicy, Warm, Aromatic, Toxic during pregnancy
HRT, SP, LIV

~ Strongly opens the orifices, revives the spirit, unblocks closed disorders
~ Invigorates the blood, dissipates clumps, reduces swelling, alleviates pain, and opens the channels

---

There was a country
whose citizens I could smell
Argentine leather

No one else could smell it
except a halfling like me

Earth and detergent
animal and Italy
and longing,,, longing

Shi Chang Pu

Sweetflag Rhizome

Rhizoma Acori Tatarinowii / Graminei

Acrid, Bitter, Warm, Aromatic
HRT, ST

~ Opens the orifices, vaporizes phlegm, quiets the spirit, removes filth, and disperses wind
~ Harmonize the middle Jiao, transform turbid damp, mobilizes the spleen and awakens the movement of QI
~ Promotes blood flow, reduces swelling, and alleviates wind damp cold
~ Benefits the throat and the voice

Knowledge cannot cure
a gutful of parasites
only wisdom can

Plants come from dirt and water
but dirt and water are not plants

Maybe that is true
But wisdom can pull the two
out of the one

Su He Xiang

Rose Maloes, Turkish Sweetgum resin
Levant Styrax

Sweet, Spicy, Warm
HRT, SP

~ Opens the orifices and penetrates through turbidity and phlegm
~ Relieves pain in the chest and abdomen, opens up stagnation, and
  clears away turbidity

On my first visit
I saw the room with my nose
and knew it to be home

My eyes were the last to see
that the windows were misplaced

Moving van driver
My wife, in a truckers cap
changes our address

Herbs That Release the Exterior Wind Cold

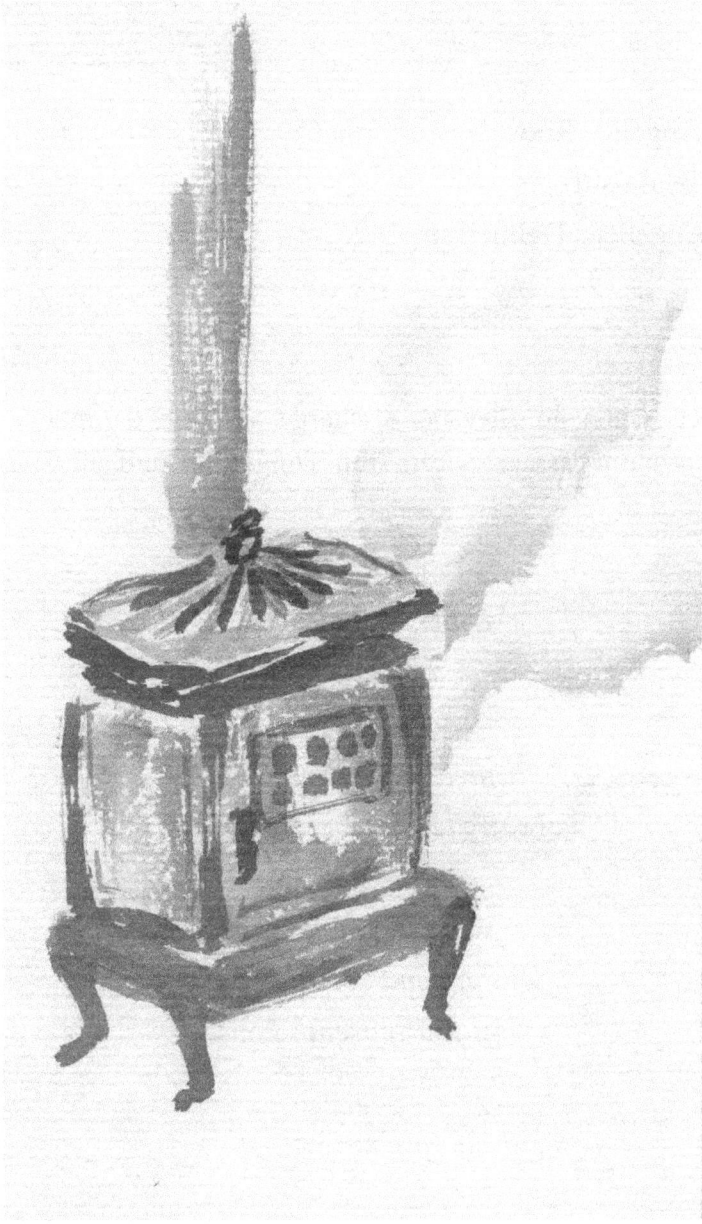

Bai Zhi

White Angelica Root
白芷 (Byakushi)
Radix Angelicae Dahuricae

Spicy, Warm
LU, SP, ST

~ Expels wind cold, alleviates discharge, and dries dampness
~ Opens nasal passages, clears sinus congestion, and alleviates pain

---

I avoid your clan
Members of your family
are truly toxic

Seated in the dining room
I can't tell doctors from death

White umbrella nurse
let's pretend you didn't grow
in your parent's house

Cong Bai

Spring Green Onion
Bulbus Allii

Spicy, Warm
LU, ST

~ Releases exterior and induces sweating
~ Disperses cold and unblocks Yang
~ Kills parasites, relieves toxins, and disperses clumps

Beaver is a fish
if you eat it on Friday
Says the Franciscan

Underneath the handkerchief
Ortolan hides from god

The monk from Thailand
Snips the greens into his soup
Ignoring the roots

Fang Feng

Laserwort, Siler, Wind-Protector Root
防風 (Bofu)
Radix Saposhnikoviae / Ledebouriellae

Acrid, Sweet, Slightly Warm
Bl, LI, LU, SP

~ Releases exterior and expels external wind
~ Helps other herbs expel wind damp, alleviates pain, and relieve spasms
~ Harmonizes spleen and liver arguments

The wall's architect
Divided the hot springs
but left thoughtful gaps

no one can directly look
even though we all want to

I cannot resist
Peeking through the windscreen gap
I see an eye!

Gao Ben

Chinese Lovage, Lugusticum Root
Rhizoma Ligustici

Spicy, Warm
BL, LIV

~ Expels wind cold in the head
~ Dispels wind and dampness

It's almost mythic
head to Root and Root to head
Chinese Lovage Root

Going to the gym today
Sculpting muscles with gazes

I touch with my eyes
long before I can listen
with my fingertips

Gui Zhi

Cassia, Cinnamon Twig
桂枝 (Keishi)
Ramulus Cinnamomi

Spicy, Sweet, Warm
BL, HRT, LU

~ Releases the exterior, assists Yang, adjusts the Ying and Wei, and releases the muscle layer
~ Assists heart Yang, resolves blood stagnation and warms the channels
~ Clears edema and accumulation of cold phlegm, unblocks Yang Qi in the chest

---

Of all his spices
the tea shaman treasured this
Cinnamon twigs

The potency remaining
from the day he plucked them

I can smell the warmth
deep in the damp of Portland
underneath the bridge

Jing Jie

Japanese Catnip
荊芥 (Keigai)
Herba Schizonepetae

Spicy, Slightly Warm, Aromatic
LIV, LU

~ Expels wind and releases the exterior
~ Resolve itching and vents rashes
~ Dispels wind and relieves muscle spasms

His name was Dickens
we found him in Christmas snow
living in a foot print

The cold was so deep in him
that he slept in the furnace

years later, sneaking in
a cat with a hole in its side
Our reputation

Ma Huang

Whorehouse Tea, Chinese Joint Fir, Mormon Tea

麻黄 (Mao)

Herbae Ephedrae

Slightly Bitter, Spicy, Warm
BL, LU

~ Induce sweating to release the exterior
~ Disperse and guides lung qi
~ Promote urination and reduces edema
~ Warms and disperses pathogenic cold

Apothecary
Treats righteous and religions
with the same herbals

Disease pays for no women
and it does not stop for church

Joy and memories
Gas station to pharmacy
Ma Huang and I

Qiang Huo

Notopterygium Root

羌活 (Kyokatsu)

Radix et Rhizoma Notopterygii

Bitter, Spicy, Warm, Aromatic
BL, KI

~ Release exterior, removes obstructions, and disperse cold, wind, and damp from the joints
~ Guides herbs into the Governing Vessel and Tai Yang channels

---

The pen doesn't guide
the senator's voting hand
Wife's perfume lingers

It is within the bedroom
that secrets and oaths are made

From the gallery
she is making sure his pen
stays loyal to her

Sheng Jiang

Fresh Ginger Root
生姜 (Shokyo)
Rhizoma Zingiberis Recens

Spicy, Slightly Warm
LU, SP, ST

~ Release the exterior, promotes perspirations, and drives out the cold
~ Warms the middle Jiao and harmonizes the stomach
~ Alleviates coughing and warms lung
~ Reduces the toxicity of other herbs

Sitting on her heels
A pile of yellow roots
Both beaming with pride

Ginger sold from the dirt road
tells its journey in flavor

Under fluorescents
it's ginger only in name
Everything else, sold

Xi Xin

Manchurian Wild Ginger

細辛 (Saishin)

Herba cum Radix Asari

Spicy, Warm, Slightly Toxic
KI, HRT, LU

~ Helps other herbs release exterior cold
~ Dispels wind and internal cold and relieves pain
~ Transforms phlegm, warms the lungs, and unblocks nasal congestion
~ Helps with oral injuries and toothache

One in the morning
the one-legged man
under the streetlight

We spilt some oranges
he tells me of his life

I give him a pack
filled with blankets, hope, and soap
and wishes and dreams

Xiang Ru

Aromatic Madder
Herba Mosiae

Spicy, Slightly Warm, Aromatic
LU, ST

~ Induces sweating, releases the exterior and, expels summer heat
~ Transforms dampness and harmonizes the spleen and stomach
~ Promotes urination and reduces swelling

In our underwear
hiding from the mid-day sun
eating Otter-Pops

Outside the grass is growing
nature will outlast us all

When the sun goes down
we take to the cul-de-sac
to soak up the night

Xin Yi Hua

Magnolia Flower Bud
Flos Magnoliae

Spicy, Warm
LU, ST

~   Expels wind cold and unblocks the sinuses

Snipping candle tips
the earthy candelabra
goes from white to brown

The Daoists say it adds ten years
I get richer by stealing

Thirty flower buds
Thirty candles on my cake
Illuminated

Zi Su Ye

Perilla Leaf
紫蘇葉 (Shisoyo)
Folium Perillae

Spicy, Warm, Aromatic
LU, SP

~ Release the exterior and disperse cold
~ Resolve qi stagnation in spleen and stomach, open chest, and calms nausea
~ Calm restless fetus and helps morning sickness

Between the needles
from the thistles and junkies
the wild plum tree

filling plastic grocery bags
Drawing looks from passers by

Wild eye wonder
why would no one else join me
in the purple rain

Herbs That Release Exterior Wind Heat

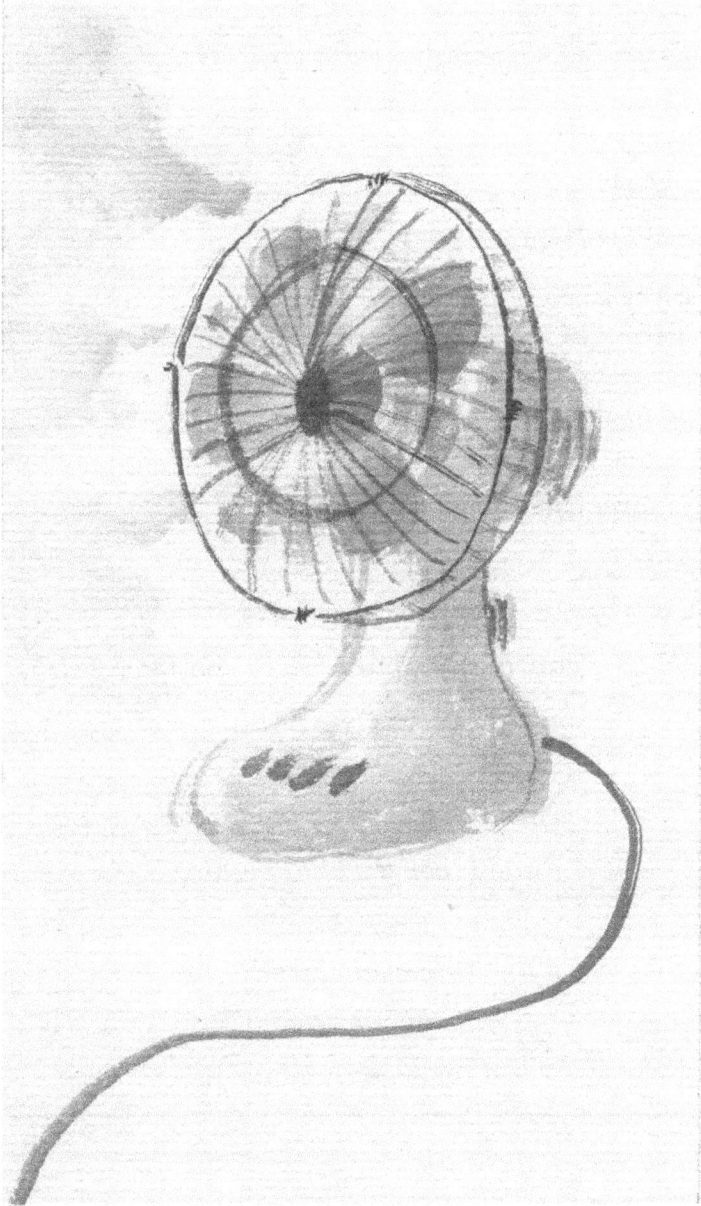

Bo He

Field Mint

薄荷 (Hakka)

Herba Menthae Haplocalycis

Spicy, Cool, Aromatic
LIV, LU

~ Expels wind heat and cools the head
~ Vents rashes and expels turbid filth
~ Resolves liver Qi Stagnation

Near the riverbank
growing fast, but without charm
tasteless river mint

The mud took one of my shoes
and I took ten of its plants

Refine and distill
Into an ounce of oil
I condense summer

Chai Hu

Hare's Ear, Bupleurum Root
柴胡 (Saiko)
Radix Bupleuri

Bitter, Spicy, Cool
GB, LIV, PC

~ Clears Shao Yang disorders, disperses wind heat and reduces fever
~ Relieves liver qi stagnation and clears emotional pain
~ Raises Yang Qi in gallbladder, spleen, and stomach deficiency
   patterns

Two arguing men
an old lady steps between
The hand of Buddha

After a night of drinking
everything is flammable

A spider web forms
Two bears fighting on a bus
Head strike the windshield

Chan Tui

Cicada molting

蝉退 (Zentai)

Periostracum Cicadae

Salty, Sweet, Cool
LU, LIV

~ Disperses wind and clears heat
~ Strongly relieves itching and vents rashes
~ Clears eyes and removes superficial visual obstructions
~ Stops spasms and extinguishes liver wind

What we leave behind
In our parents basements
Photos and moltings?

Stashed in a wood speaker
angry rambling and ------

In a box somewhere
Is my keychain collection
and hope, endless hope

Dan Dou Chi

Prepared Fermented Soybean
Semen Sojae Preparatum

Sweet, Slightly Bitter, Cold
LU, ST

~ Releases both exterior hot or cold (depending on how it is prepared)
~ Eliminates irritability, restlessness, insomnia, and harmonizes the middle Jiao
~ Clears fire, settles Qi, and eliminates damp heat

At the front counter
a customer brings me a gift
of fermented beans

Blind myself from co-workers
whose eyes sparkle with judgment

For just a moment
we both ignore social norms
and I accept it

Fu Ping

Duckweed
Herba Spirodelae

Spicy, Cool
BL, LU

~ Clears exterior heat, induces sweating, and promotes urination
~ Unblocks the muscle layer and vents rashes

Winged inkblots diving
black and white became green
duckweed in the pond

I wait for him to surface
Anxious, in nature's flawed way

Car crosses the bridge
Radio blares like Thisby
Panic from a Prius

Ge Gen

Kudzu Root
葛根 (Kakkon)
Radix Puerariae

Sweet, Spicy, Cool
SP, ST

~ Releases upper muscles, clears heat, and discharges exterior
  conditions
~ Nourishes the fluids and alleviates thirst, and alleviates diarrhea

---

Giving and giving
Stopping panic, choking panic
Giving and giving

Excess becomes deficient
Binding becomes strangling

When mud starts to creep
and all one has is kindness,
talk to the devil

Ju Hua

Chrysanthemum flower
菊花 (Kikuja)
Flos Chrysanthemi

Sweet, Bitter, Cool
LIV, LU

~ Disperses wind and clears heat
~ Clears liver and the eyes
~ Calms liver Yang and extinguishes wind
~ Promotes the movement of heart Qi, detoxifies and stimulates the
  blood

Growing in planters
Mums at the light rail stop
I pluck it with my teeth

Before the sun rises
I look to brighten my eyes

Later I find out
what I ate was not what I thought
but what I needed

Man Jing Zi

Vitex, Chaste Tree Fruit
蔓荆子 (Mankeishi)
Fructus Viticis

Bitter, Cool
BL, LIV, ST

~ Disperses wind and clears heat
~ Clears wind heat in the liver channel
~ Drains dampness, expels wind, and relieves pain

A moment, alone
A monk thinks of younger days
fingers his prayer beads

nearby, a dish is served
"Buddha jumps over the wall"

he gets on his knees
What erodes him when held in
erodes him when let out

Mu Zei

Horse-Tail, Shave Grass
Herba Equiseti Hiemalis

Bitter, Sweet, Neutral
LIV, LU

~ Disperses wind heat and eliminates superficial visual obstruction
~ Clears heat and stops bleeding

Doctor's once told me
That four seeds destroy synapse
god, I hope they're right

A gift of herbs meant to heal
Powerless before chemistry

Science poisons me
and there is no antidote
Knowledge's venom

Niu Bang Zi

Arctium, Great Burdock Fruit

牛蒡子 (Goboshi)

Fructus Arctii

Bitter, Spicy, Cool
LU, ST

~ Disperses wind heat and benefits throat
~ Relieves toxicity and encourages rashes
~ Moistens the intestines and clears wind heat toxins

Red plastic baskets
Colliding in the produce
Apples and pears watch

The gaijin and obasan
exchanging bows and smiles

she points at "aperu"
"ReIngou dezu kA?"
"Ah! Jozu dess!"

Sang Ye

White Mulberry Leaf
桑葉 (Soyo)
Folium Mori

Bitter, Sweet, Cold
LIV, LU

~ Clears lung heat and moistens dryness
~ Cools liver and clears the eyes
~ Cools the blood, disperses wind heat, and stops bleeding

Carry some tissues
It's a gift we all will need
but we never want

A symbol of weaknesses
that we could all do without

I wipe my nose
and everything falls apart
Blood, snot, and tears

Sheng Ma

Black Cohosh

升麻 (Shoma)

Rhizoma Cimicifugae

Spicy, Sweet, Slightly Cold
LI, LU, SP, ST

~ Releases the exterior and vents early measles
~ Clears heat and relieves toxicity
~ Raises Yang, boosts heart Yin, and lifts spleen Qi sinking
~ Helps guide other herbs upwards

A clean bill of health
for herself, and no one else
Crisis averted

Everyone has accidents
but she won't be one of them

So liberating
To finally be in control
of Destiny's horse

Herbs That Relieve Coughing and Wheezing

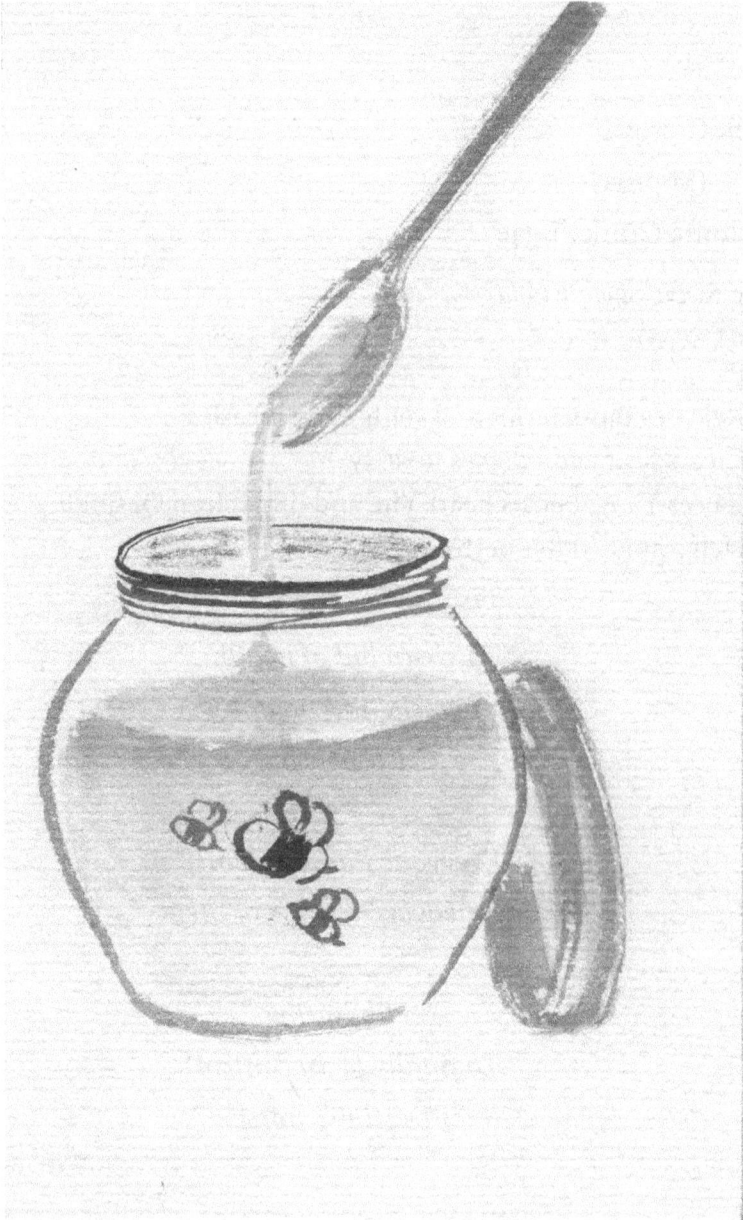

Bai Bu

Stemona Root
Radix Stemonae

Bitter, Sweet, Slightly Warm
LU

~   Moistens the lungs and stops cough
~   Expels parasites and kills bugs

Reading Kerouak
A bug crawls across my foot
I hesitate ---

This wouldn't be the first book
that impressed a bug

We laugh at the pun
It continues on its way
And its eaten by the cat

Kuan Dong Hua

Tussilago, Coltsfoot Flower

款冬花 (Kantoka)

Flos Farfarae

Spicy, Warm
LU

~ Moistens the lungs, transforms phlegm, stops cough, and redirects qi downward

---

On my teacher's desk
stickers, hand sanitizer
photos of her kids

She remembered my first work
"Construction-Paper-Watermelon"

She mentions my name
I'm filled with the same pride
I had when I was seven

Ma Dou Ling

Dutchman's Pipe Fruit
Fructus Aristolochiae

Bitter, Slightly Cold
LI, LU

~ Clears the lungs, transforms phlegm, and stops coughing and wheezing
~ Clears and drains large intestine heat and reduces swelling and pain

---

A Marlboro man
to American Spirit
Lung cancer branding

For the good times and bad times
two lighter strikes and a puff

An honest question:
Are the lost moments as good
as the ones smoked?

Meng Shi

Mica, Chlorite
Lapis Chloriti

Salty, Sweet, Neutral
LI, LU, ST

~ Directs qi downward and reduces phlegm
~ Calms the liver and suppresses convulsions

Jewelry becomes cheap
only when we decide
that it should be cheap

A pewter charm from the fair
as precious as my wedding band

There once was a clan
who hid rubies in their skin
for divine blessings

Mu Hu Die / Gui Zhi Hua

Oroxylum Seeds
Semen Oroxyli

Bland, Sweet, Cool
LIV, LU

~ Moistens the lungs and clears and the voice
~ Comforts the liver and regulates Qi
~ Promotes healing of damp heat ulcers in the skin

Once while being mugged
and once as a soloist
Two times terrified

No amount of applauding
could cure me of stage fright

And yet I went out
Belting bravery over fear
Clad in Fagan's rag

Pi Pa Ye

Loquat Leaf
枇杷葉 (Biwayo)
Folium Eriobotryae

Bitter, Neutral
LU, ST

~ Transforms phlegm, clears lung heat, and guides lung Qi down
~ Harmonizes the stomach, clears stomach heat, and guides stomach Qi down

---

Who were you drawn for
Cartoon on the couch syrup
Parent or child

Making light of vicious croup
Reminding "This too shall pass"

Stressful week passes
Having drinks with a mascot
Codeine cocktail

Sang Bai Pi

White Mulberry Root Bark

桑白皮 (sohakuhi)

Cortex Mori

Sweet, Cold
LU

~ Drains lung heat and stops coughing and wheezing
~ Promotes urination and reduces edema

I trip on a root
And then spent the next hour
tripping on the root

It was a nice day, I assume
My phone flying, then cracking

The song birds singing
and all I can think about
are my mp3s

Su Zi

Perilla Fruit
Fructus Perillae

Spicy, Warm
LI, LU

~ Stops coughing and wheezing, dissolves phlegm, and guides the Qi
 downward
~ Moistens the intestines and unblock the bowel

Panicked, he called me
"I caught IT… in my zipper"
and I need your help!

Yunnan's White Medicine
and needle-nose pliers

Bleeding and screaming
Then Bai Yao and blowing air
An awkward first date

Ting Li Zi

Wood Whitlow Grass, Tingli Seed
Semen Lepidii / Descurainiae

Spicy, Bitter, Very Cold
BL, LU

~   Drains lung heat, reduces phlegm, and calms wheezing
~   Churns the water and reduces edema

I once knew a girl
who stung those closest to her
whose name meant honey

Others would disapprove
when, twice stung, I would swat

"Can you blame a bee
with honeycomb in her heart?
It's in her nature"

Xing Ren

Bitter Apricot kernel
杏仁 (Kyonin)
Semen Armeniacae

Bitter, Slightly Warm, Slightly Toxic
LI, LU

~ Stops cough and calms wheezing
~ Moistens the intestines and unblocks the bowels.

I knew another:
As sweet as an apricot
with a bitter core

Tossed the fruit and cracked the shell
I reveled in its bitterness

Treasure surrounding
Sitting amongst the shells
A shit-eating grin

Zi Wan

Purple Aster Root
Radix Asteris

Bitter, Spicy, Slightly Warm
LU

~   Relieves cough and expels phlegm

Empty looking house
An ancient hands us apples
Our parents don't trust

We are taught to believe
that strangers are dangerous

For 13 years
we take her apple slices
Every Halloween

Herbs That Relieve Food Stagnation

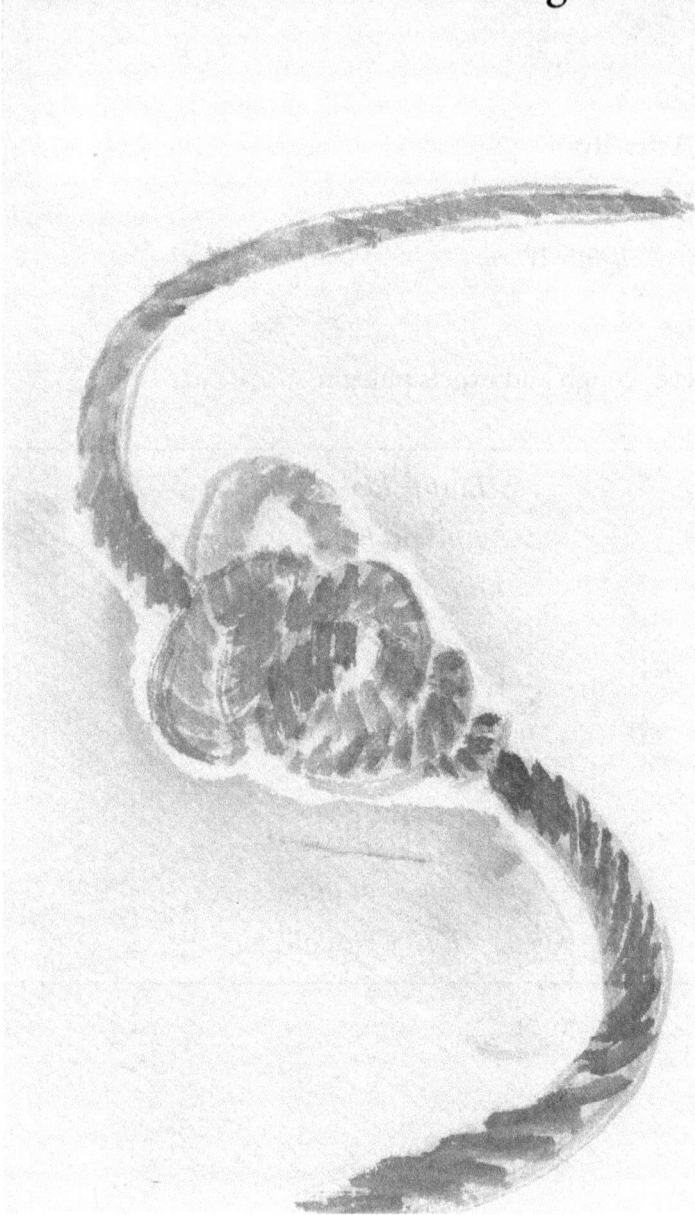

Gu Ya / Su Ya

Millet or Rice sprouts

Fructus Setariae Germinatus

Fructus Oryzae Germinatus

Sweet, Warm
SP, ST

~ Reduces food stagnation, strengthens the stomach, and
  harmonizes the center
~ Strengthens the Spleen and encourages the appetite

The first time I bought
a 20 lb bag of rice
I was my proudest

What child would buy that much?
Independent men buy rice

I burnt the first pot
and the second was bitter
Both tasted the best

Ji Nei Jin

Chicken Gizzard lining
Endothelium Corneum Gigeriae Galli

Sweet, Neutral
BL, SI, SP, ST

~ Strongly reduces food stagnation and strengthen the transport function of the spleen
~ Secures the Jing and stops enuresis
~ Transforms hardness and dissolves stones

They have no morals
Nor qualms with ending a life
Towering emus

Ones head got stuck in a fence
And ripped off in a panic

Throat, a booming drum
Its eggs, giant drops of jade
God's sense of humor

Lai Fu Zi

Radish Seed
Semen Raphani

Spicy, Sweet, Neutral
LU, SP, ST

~ Reduces food stagnation, transforms accumulations, promotes
 digestion, and reduces distention
~ Descends lung qi and reduces phlegm

All summer we pulled
radish after radish up
from our square of dirt

They tasted like sunshine
and tingled like a sunburn

I've never tasted
another quite like those ones
we grew without growing

Mai Ya

Malt, Barley Sprouts
Fructus Hordei Germinatus

Sweet, Neutral
LIV, SP, ST

~ Reduces food stagnation, improves digestion, and strengthens the
  stomach
~ Smoothes the flow of liver Qi

The lawnmower man
left a stand of false nettles
by the Aspen tree

He eats his home-packed lunch
near the fruits of his mercy

His sharp purple hope.
The remainder of the yard
trimmed to an inch

Shan Zha

Mountain Hawthorn Fruit

山楂子 (Sanzashi)

Fructus Crataegi

Sour, Sweet, Slightly Warm
LIV, SP, ST

~ Reduces and moves food stagnation and accumulations out
~ Transforms blood stasis, dissipates clumps, and invigorates the blood.
~ Stops diarrhea

I eat a haw disk
and hope to gain the beauty
of the spokesmodel

With fox nuts and gou qi zi
Dispensary trail mix

When did I give up
buckets of reality
for pre-packed promises

Shen Qu

Massa Fermentata, Medicated Leaven
Massa Medicata Fermentata

Spicy, Sweet, Warm
SP, ST

~ Reduces food stagnation, moves Qi, strengthens the stomach, and
  promotes digestion

Take everything good
and press it into a brick

Massa fermenta
It was a tangle of things
Now, It's its own medicine

Massa fermenta
I asked what it was made of
"Massa fermenta"

Herbs That Stabilize and Bind

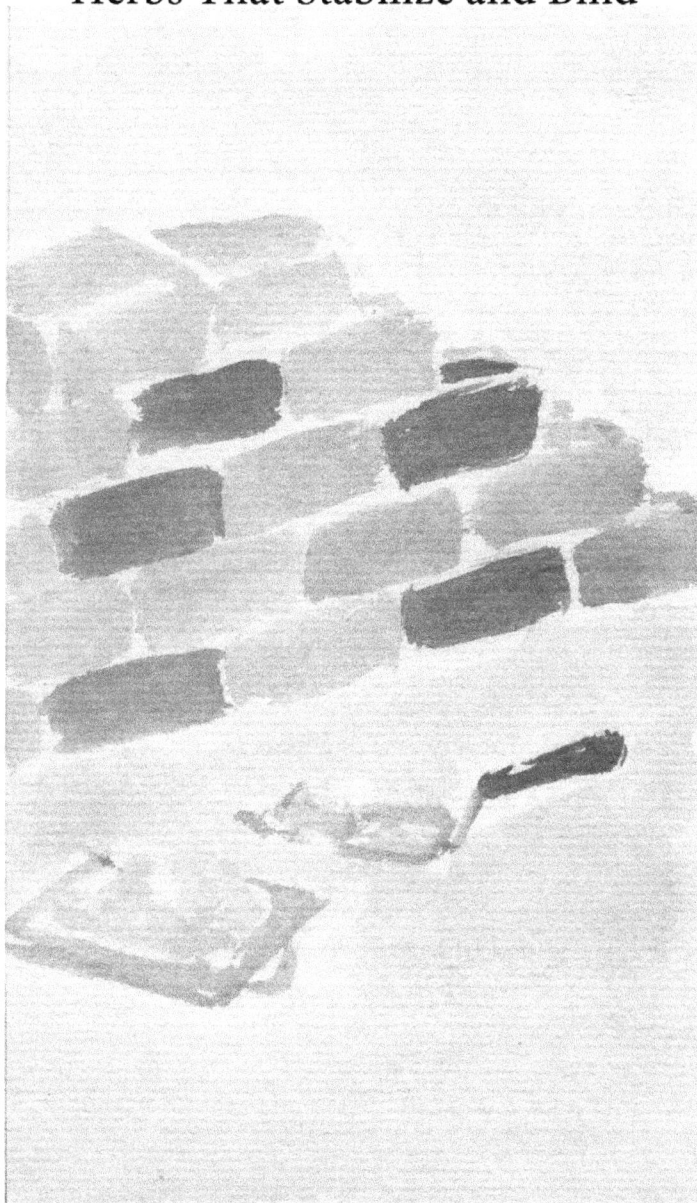

Bai Guo

Ginko Nut
Semen Ginkgonis Bilobae

Astringent, Bitter, Sweet, Neutral, Slightly Toxic
LU

~ Nourish the lungs and stop wheezing
~ Eliminate dampness, stop discharges, and stabilizes the lower Jiao

---

Amongst the gold
treasure for squirrel and scholar
A pearl of sweet wood

Someone said it was toxic
Knowledge can feel that way

A rock striking wood
What I thought was enlightenment
makes my dentist rich

Chi Shi Zhi

Red Halloysite, Red Kaolin
Halloysitum Rubrum

Astringent, Sour, Sweet, Warm
LI, SP, ST

~ Holds the intestines, stops cold diarrhea
~ Contain the blood and stop bleeding
~ Promotes healing of wounds and generates flesh

Eating spicy food
Consequences today
Also tomorrow

A child with a pop-gun
A mild habanero

All over the world
We chase poison with poison
Life's celebration

Chun Pi

Tree of Heaven Bark
Cortex Ailanthi

Astringent, Bitter, Cold
LI, ST

~ Clears heat, dries dampness, astringes the intestines, and stops
  leakage in the lower Jiao
~ Kills parasites and scabies

Climbing to heaven
Take a break in the branches
And chew on the Bark

We are given five senses
To delight God with stories

First one I will tell:
The story of finding you
and losing myself

Fu Pen Zi

Chinese Raspberry Fruit
Fructus Rubi

Astringent, Sweet, Neutral
KI, LIV

~ Tonifies and stabilizes the kidney Qi, binds the Jing, and restrains urine
~ Tonifies Yang and improves vision

Here a "noxious weed"
In the East, the prince of fruit
Chinese Raspberry

A tyrant who conquers the land
A leader that gives to all

Tamed by plastic
You become a figurehead
living in exile

Fu Xiao Mai

Wheat Berry
Fructus Tritici Levis

Sweet, Slightly Salty, Cool
HRT

~   Stops excessive sweating from deficiency
~   Nourish the heart and calms the spirit

On the Kansas plain
Blue-white sky and khaki land
Winter wheat harvest

The sound of silence
The sound of wheatstraw

My heart goes fallow
Stupid habits and vices
Tilled into soil

Hai Piao Xiao

Cuttlefish Bone

Endoconcha Sepiae

Astringent, Salty, Slightly Warm
KI, LIV, ST

~ Retains Jing due to kidney deficiency
~ Harmonizes the stomach, controls acidity, resolves dampness, and
   promotes healing

It's not bitter
That keeps me away from you
It's the stink

What fetid mass grows in you
Leaves slicks of odor on me

I'm not popular
But hanging around with you
I see their noses turn

He Zi

Myrobalan Fruit

訶子 (Kashi)

Fructus Chebulae

Astringent, Bitter, Sour, Neutral
LI, LU, ST

~ Binds and astringes the intestines
~ Contains lung Qi leakage, stops cough, wheezing, and loss of voice

---

Segment by segment
Juicy cell by juicy cell
I eat the orange

An intimate food affair
I consume it forever

Strange eyes and words
No one appreciates
the effort of Life

Jin Ying Zi

Cherokee Rose Hip
Fructus Rosae Laevigatae

Sour, Neutral
BL, KI, LI

~   Stabilize the kidneys, retains Jing, and astringes urine
~   Binds the intestines and stops diarrhea

A woman who crosses
the prairie's barbed fences
wearing rose petals

She draws no property lines
and commits no trespassing

Painful to forage
Yet the thought of uprooting
is much more painful

Lian Zi

Lotus Seed
蓮子 (Renshi)
Semen Nelumbinis

Astringent, Sweet, Neutral
HRT, KI, SP

~ Tonifies the spleen and stops diarrhea
~ Tonifies the kidneys and stabilize Jing
~ Nourish the heart, calms the spirit, and flushes irritability

---

Growing from the mud
in the pure lotus wisdom
lies a simple food

The true gift of the dharma
is the gift of giving

At the Great Lecture
he showed us all a flower
and we all ate the seeds

Ma Huang Gen

Ephedra Root
Radix Ephedrae

Sweet, Neutral
LU

~ Stops sweat due to deficiency
~ Known to reverse effects of Ma Huang

A plant with 2 names
Apprentice Stem, Master's Root
spirit and knowledge

One found in truck stops
The other in textbooks

We all start somewhere
and after reaching upwards
end where we begin

Nuo Dao Gen Xu

Glutinous Rice Root

Radix Oryzae Glutinosae

Sweet, Neutral
KI, LI, LU

~ Stops sweating caused by deficiency and increases saliva
~ Clears deficient Yin fevers

Kimono in public
The most judgmental glances
Come from the mirror

A star thinks it's the brightest
amongst its billion brothers

Accessorizing:
Confidence would look the best
but it doesn't fit

Qian Shi

Foxnut

Semen Euryales

Astringent, Sweet, Neutral
KI, SP

- ~ Strengthen spleen and stop diarrhea.
- ~ Stabilize kidneys and retains kidney Jing
- ~ Expels dampness and stops discharge

Happy birthday fox!
You came into my world
30 years ago

I left you nuts and saké
underneath the hemlock

Follow me around
and show me pretty things
under the sun

Rou Dou Kou

Nutmeg
Semen Myristicae

Spicy, Warm
LU, SP, ST

~ Dries the intestines and stops chronic diarrhea
~ Warms the middle Jiao, moves Qi, and alleviates abdominal pain

---

In selling my home
I spray the scent of nutmeg
Seeding memories

I never wanted to leave
I never wanted to stay

A couple comes in
Pregnant with child
Pregnant with hope

Shan Zhu Yu

Cornelian Cherry Fruit
山茱萸 (Sanshuyu)
Fructus Corni

Sour, Slightly Warm
KI, LIV

~ Stabilize the kidneys and retain the Jing and fluids
~ Tonifies the liver and kidney Yin and kidney Yag
~ Stabilize menses, stops excessive sweating, and supports
   devastated Yang and Qi

Out of lunch money
A fresh bag of Shan Zhu Yu
weighs a little light

Restocking the medicine
Curing my aching stomach

My palm holds a meal
7 assorted dry nuts
5 or 6 red fruits

Wu Bei Zi

Chinese Sumac gallnut

五倍子 (Gobaishi)

Galla Chinensis

Sour, Salty, Cold
KI, LI, LU

~ Contain leakage of lung Qi and stops coughing
~ Astringes the intestines, restrains leakage, and stops diarrhea
~ Absorbs moisture, reduces swelling, and relieves fire toxicity
  topically

In an Irish pub
a trio in the basement
swirls around in smoke

Faces amongst the leather
lit by embers and cell phones

A port and a pen
The last time I touched those
was when I was 12

Wu Mei

Mume Fruit
Fructus Mume

Astringent, Sour, Warm
LI, LIV, LU, SP

~ Inhibits the leakage of lung Qi, and stops sweating and coughs
~ Generates fluids, alleviates thirst, and astringes the intestines
~ Expels roundworm, and stops bleeding

Big man in purple
Tosses the troublemakers
with only his eyes

"Sir," in a baritone voice
The drunkard becomes sober

Yellow downward light
The snow drawing white angles
Sentry in a suit

Wu Wei Zi

Five-Flavor Berry, Schisandra Fruit
Fructus Schisandrae

Sour, Sweet, Warm
HRT, KI, LU

~ Constrains leakage of lung qi and enriches kidney Yin
~ Tonifies the kidneys, binds the essence, and stops diarrhea
~ Inhibits sweating and generates fluids
~ Quiets the spirit, calms the heart, and clears irritability

---

Red cup of nectar
floating from sunny to cold
Social butterfly

From Yeats to Pokemon
a collection of knowledge

The end of the night
A jug of filtered water
and a Netflix binge

Herbs That Stop Bleeding

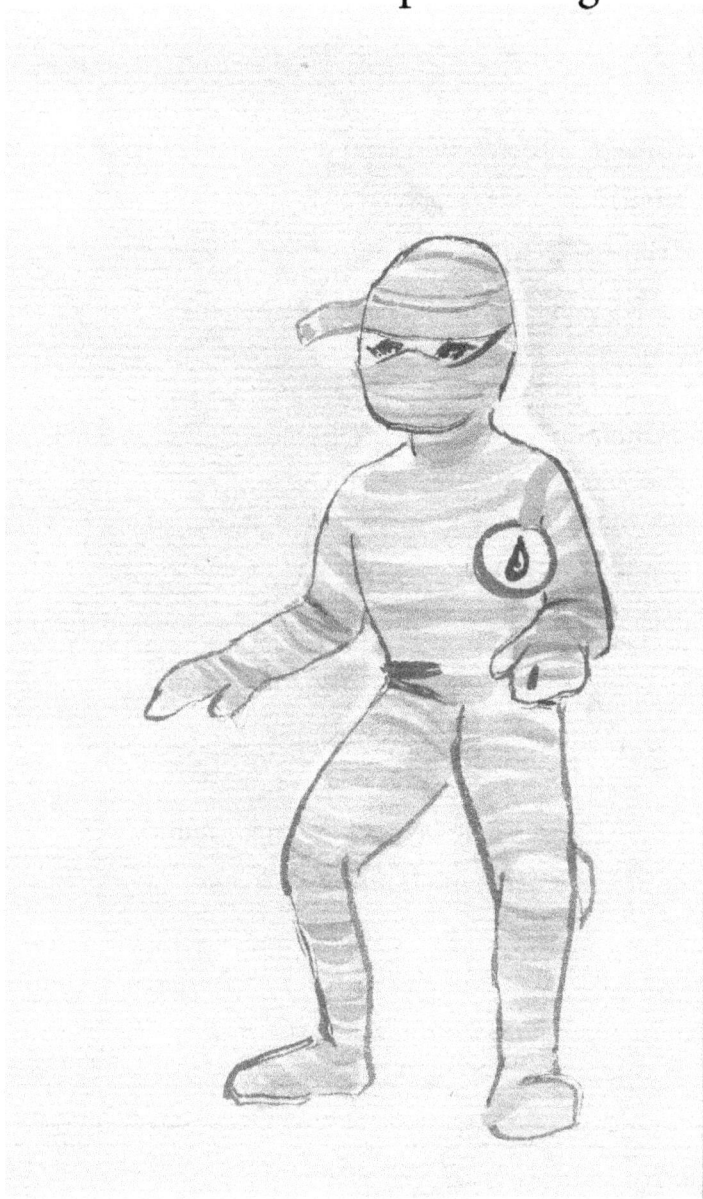

Ai Ye

Mugwort, Argyi Wormwood Leaf
艾葉 (Gaiyo)
Folium Artemisiae Argyi

Bitter, Spicy, Warm
KI, LIV, SP

~ Warms the womb, stops bleeding, and pacifies the fetus
~ Disperses cold and alleviates pain
~ Dries dampness and stops itching

In a foil wad
Smoldering white and green
Bundle of mugwort

Smoking behind the high school
we cough on an ashy high

None of us feel much
but we dream of the future
in Technicolor

Bai Ji

Bletilla Root
Rhizoma Bletillae

Astringent, Bitter, Sweet, Slightly Cold
LU, ST, LIV

~   Stops bleeding from the lungs and stomach
~   Reduces swelling and generates flesh topically

Red on my knuckles
I hope we can be friends
when he stops bleeding

Drop to the floor and lock eyes
We laugh, crimson spittle flies

Onlooker's chagrin
Embarrassed at their bloodlust
Unsure shuffling

Bai Mao Gen

White Grass Root
Rhizoma Imperatae

Sweet, Cold
LU, SI, ST

~   Cools blood and stops bleeding
~   Clears heat and promotes urination
~   Clears heat from the stomach and lungs

Mowing in patterns
for angels and airliners
to appreciate

In the summer, cut the grass
In the winter, shovel snow

Sitting in the art
Listen to dry wild straw
Listen to flakes

Ce Bai Ye

Arborvitae Leaf Tips

柏葉 (Sokuhakuyo)

Cacumen Biotae

Astringent, Bitter, Slightly Cold
LI, LIV, LU

~ Cools blood and stops bleeding
~ Stops cough, expels phlegm, and soothes asthma
~ Clears damp heat and wind dampness
~ Promote healing of burns topically

The hair club for men;
"We are all embarrassed
by what nature did"

Nothing makes one look as old
as trying to look too young

Brass nails and lasers
The pain of embarrassment
Seems not as painful

Da Ji

Japanese Thistle
Herba Sive Radix Cirsii Japonici

Sweet, Cool
HRT, LIV, SP

~ Cools the blood and stops bleeding
~ Reduces swelling, generates flesh, and moves blood stasis
~ Improves the gallbladder and reduces jaundice

The coffee shop wasp
asks me how to say phrases
like "let's run away"

I'm only a substitute
The words are for her teacher

She takes all the words;
Tossing withered embryos
at potent expats

Di Yu

Burnet-Bloodwort Root
Radix Sanguisorbae

Bitter, Sour, Slightly Cold
LI, LIV, ST

~ Cools the blood and stops bleeding
~ Clears heat, astringes the fluids, and generates flesh

In the back closet
Cheap pants and lost clothing
for poorer students

Instantly my heart drops-
Aware of battles not fought

Hormones gone jaded
But just for an instant
I become human

Huai Hua Mi

Japanese Pagoda Tree Bud
Flos Sophorae Immaturus

Bitter, Cool
LI, LIV

~   Cools the blood and stops bleeding
~   Cools the liver and clears the head

Amateur birdhouse
Perfect in its disrepair
Nobody moves in

Windstorm; it falls off its post
Crack like an egg, nest inside

A little bigger
Rebuilt in the same style
but without the leaks

Jiang Xiang

Scented Rosewood

Lignum Acronychiae

Spicy, Sweet, Warm
LIV, SP, ST

~ Disperses blood stasis and stops bleeding
~ Invigorates the blood, promotes the movement of Qi, and softens
  pain

Nothing heals faster
Than a bandage placed by mom
And sealed with a kiss

No opiate can compare
Loving eyes and a smile

Splinters to concussions
All injuries felt the same
when I ran to her

Ou Jie

Lotus Rhizome Node
Nodus Nelumbo Nuciferae

Astringent, Sweet, Neutral
LIV, LU, ST

~ Stops bleeding, breaks up blood stasis, and astringes leakage
~ Clears heat from the blood

How many chapters
and how many memories
fill your library?

Did you read all of these books
or are they just for looks

Great halls of records
Held up by fleshy synapses
designed to fail

Pu Huang

Cattail Pollen
Pollen Typhae

Spicy, Sweet, Neutral
HRT, LIV, SP

~ Stops bleeding, invigorates the blood, dispels blood stasis, and
promotes urination

Lances in the marsh
Child warriors pluck them
and fight while laughing

An explosion of cotton
the bout is decided

We battled at dusk
Any other time of day
seemed inappropriate

Qian Cao Gen

Heart-Leaf Madder Root
Radix Rubiae

Bitter, Cold
HRT, LIV

~ Cools the blood and the liver, transforms phlegm, and stops
  bleeding
~ Invigorates blood to dispel blood stasis
~ Disperses wind dampness, unblocks the channels

On the football field
you wrapped me in a blanket
and stared at the stars

It was nearly 10pm
The curfew of youth was due

Always in my trunk
I carry a time machine:
A quilted blanket

San Qi / Tian Qi

Notoginseng, Three-Seven Root
Radix Pseudoginseng

Sweet, Slightly Bitter, Warm
LIV, ST

~ Stops bleeding and transforms blood stasis
~ Alleviate pain, reduce swelling from injury, stops bleeding, and
  invigorates the blood

Energy not energy
Cans of enthusiasm
Piled in the trash

They say those drinks will kill me
Horse doesn't die from the whip

On Monday morning
there's no need to check my mood
Three half-empty mugs

Xian He Cao

Furry Agrimony
Herba Agrimoniae

Bitter, Neutral
LIV, LU, SP

~ Astringes and stops bleeding, reduces swelling, and eliminates pus
~ Kills parasites, and alleviates diarrhea and dysentery.
~ Tonifies the Qi an blood

With no one around
nostalgic stories with friends
I'm watching re-runs

Homer and I share a beer
while our respective Marges groan

Holding memories;
I'm not reading the chapter
I'm leaving bookmarks

Zi Zhu

Beauty-berry Leaf
Folium Calicarpae Formosanae

Astringent, Bitter, Cool
LIV, LU, ST

~ Stops bleeding, resolves toxicity, and treats burns and sores

---

Presenting my work
All I am thinking about
are my mis-matched socks

I believe in my research
but not my fashion senses

I come back to life
From behind the podium
no one sees my socks

Zong Lu Pi

Chinese Palm Fiber
Fibra Stipulae Trachycarpi

Bitter, Neutral
LI, LIV, LU

~ Binds leakage and stops bleeding

Twining newspaper
into colorful garlands
of unread words

Advertisers and authors
celebrating my birthday

Thrown into a bin
Back to the recycling
we all came from

Herbs That Tonifies Blood

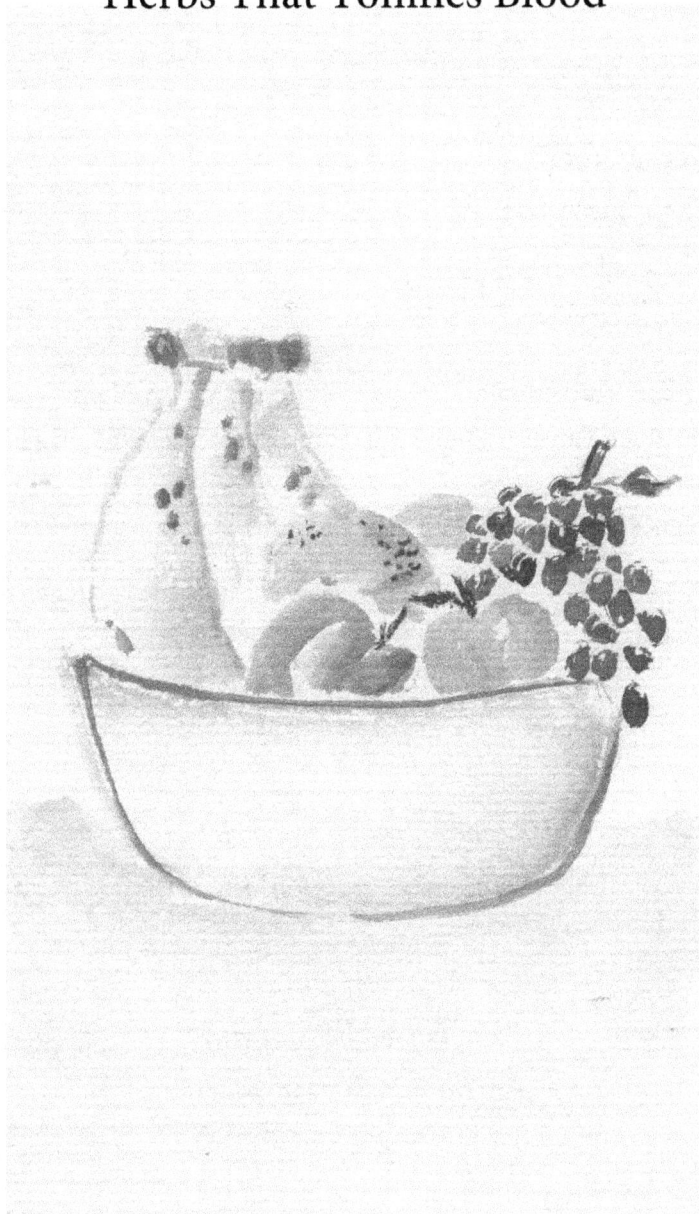

Bai Shao Yao

White Peony Root
Radix Paeoniae Alba

Bitter, Sour, Cool
LIV, SP

~ Nourishes the blood and regulates menstrual problems
~ Calms liver Yang and wind, alleviates pain, and alleviates liver Qi issues
~ Preserves Yin and adjusts Ying and Wei levels

Slices from the white
Delicately on my tongue
Cooling my liver

On the wall of miracles
Stood out, a bump in the air

Aspect of a nurse
Calm voiced bedside angel
Simple Root slices

Dang Gui

Chinese Angelica Root

当帰 (Toki)

Radix Angelicae Sinensis

Bitter, Sweet, Pungent, Warm
HRT, LIV, SP

~ Tonifies the blood and regulates menstruation
~ Invigorates and harmonizes the blood, disperses cold, and stops stasis pain
~ Moistens dry intestines and loosens the bowels
~ Reduces swellings, expels pus, and generates flesh

Eyes, thrusting at me
She asks me to save something
Papers thrust at me

There are still those who believe
before the world dries them out

From souls to soldiers
Without a cash donation
nothing is saved?

E Jiao

Donkey-Hide Gelatin
阿膠 (Akyo)
Gelatinum Corii Asini

Sweet, Neutral
KI, LIV, LU

~ Tonifies and nourishes the blood, and stops bleeding
~ Nourish the Yin and moisten the lungs and large intestine

Bricks like Latinum
A foul tasting medicine
stacked like bullion

Both have their roots in stories
Legendary currency

E Jiao and raw eggs
Morning after the concert
I pay my debt twice

Gou Qi Zi

Chinese Wolfberry, Matrimony Vine, Lycium Fruit

枸杞子 (Kukoshi)

Fructus Lycii

Sweet, Neutral
KI, LIV, LU

~ Nourishes and tonifies liver and kidney Yin and blood
~ Benefits Jing and brightens the eyes
~ Enriches Yin and moistens the lungs

My friends know you as
"A medicated raisin
that benefits all"

For one with so many names
that is the greatest title

No hidden meaning
Just the truth in plain language
Anyone could grasp

He Shou Wu

Mr. He's Black Hair, Flowery Knotweed Root

何首烏 (Kashu)

Radix Polygoni Multiflori Preparata

Astringent, Bitter, Sweet, Slightly Warm
KI, LIV

~ Tonifies liver and kidney, nourishes blood, and boosts the Jing
~ Relieves toxic fire and expels wind from the skin
~ Moistens intestines and unblock the bowel

Each hair that fell out
A transgression reminder
With vanity pain

From below a reminder
But from above, a promise

Angels pluck away
Until I look less manly
and more like a monk

Long Yan Rou

Dragon's Eye, Longan Fruit
竜眼肉 (Ryuganniku)
Arillus Longan

Sweet, Warm
HRT, SP

~ Tonifies the heart and spleen, nourishes blood, and calms the
  spirit

The Eye of Taurus
Watches over laborers
of body and soul

Smokey "Dragon Eye" Longan
works calmly without stressing

There are much worse fates
than to suffer the hardship
of good works given to us

Shu Di Huang

Prepared Chinese Foxglove Root
Radix Rehmanniae Preparata

Sweet, Slightly Warm
HRT, KI, LIV

~ Tonifies and nourishes the blood, the liver, and kidney Yin
~ Strongly nourishes the Yin, Jing, and blood, fills the marrow, and
stops lower Jiao wasting

Mashed and cooked
improves marrow and the brain
looking like what it treats

Only the Most Inspired
would leave us such careful clues

In the north and south
from the far east to the west
Like cures Like

Sang Shen

Mulberry Fruit
Fructus Mori

Sweet, Cold
HRT, KI, LIV

~   Tonifies blood and enriches Yin
~   Lubricates the intestines and generates fluids

At the bodega
A box of mulberry fruit
A can of Vimto

Sitting in the parking lot
Mixing unknown with unknown

In a German car
J-pop and Turkish candy
Enjoying the sun

Herbs That Tonifies Qi

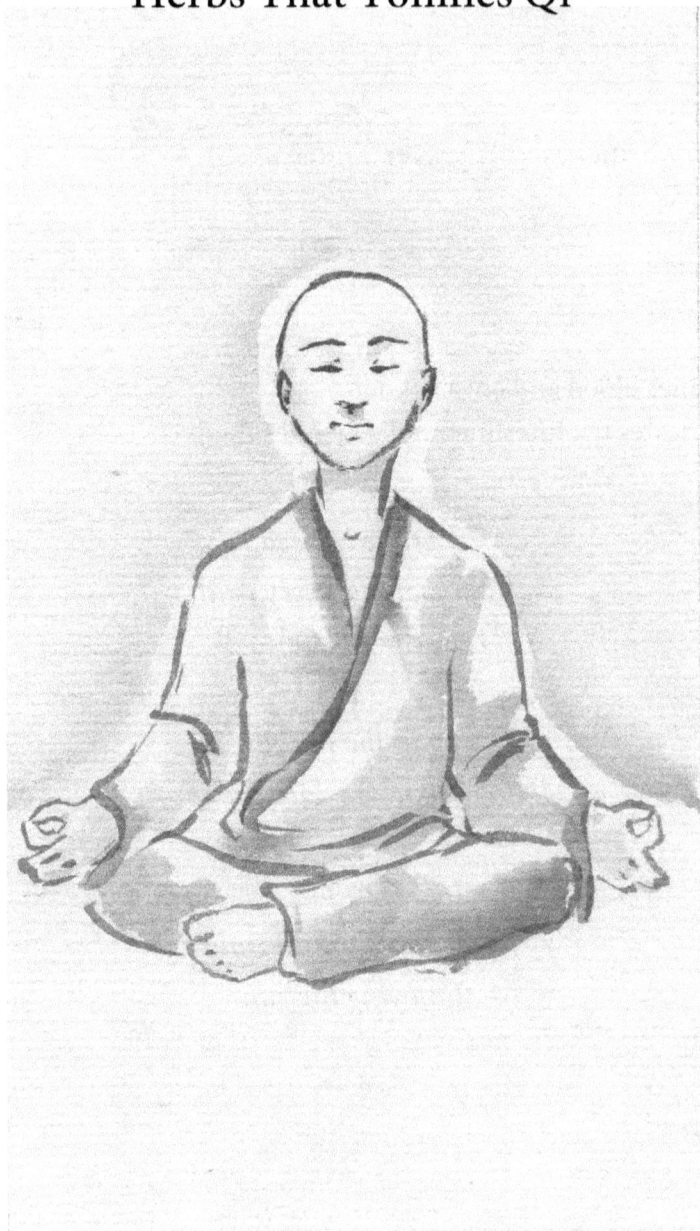

Bai Zhu

White Atractylodis Rhizome
白芷 (Byakushi)
Rhizoma Atractylodis Macrocephalae

Bitter, Sweet, Warm
SP, ST

~ Tonifies the spleen and augments qi
~ Stabilizes the exterior and stops sweating
~ Dries dampness and retains moisture

Pairing cheese and tea
We taste one and then another
Do plum and hay mix?

Two masters of the tongue
Paint portraits of sheep and hills

The tea maker sells
Half the flavor for the mouth
and half for the ears

Da Zao

Jujube Berry
大棗 (Taiso)
Fructus Jujube

Sweet, Warm
SP, ST

~ Tonifies spleen and stomach Qi
~ Nourishes the blood and calms the spirit
~ Softens the negative effects of other herbs

Hold it, sweetly.
Refrain from biting too deep
or you'll find, the pit

I shove it all in my mouth
and let my teeth sort it out

Sweetness bound to stone
Flesh bound to the skeleton
Green bound to the Earth

Dang Shen

Codonopsis Root
Radix Codonopsis

Sweet Neutral
LU, SP

~ Tonifies the middle Jiao and augments the QI
~ Tonifies the lungs
~ Nourishes the body and generates fluids
~ Often used with herbs that release the exterior when patient has significant qi deficiency.

Red satin curtains
over white venetian blinds
filtering sunrise

Wrapped in the dough of my bed
my room becomes an oven

After the sunset
In rows across my bedspread
slats of moonlight fall

Gan Cao

Licorice Root

甘草 (Kanzo)

Radix Glycyrrhizae

Sweet, Neutral
HRT, LU, SP ST

~ Tonifies the spleen and augments Qi
~ Remedies Qi and blood deficiency with irregular pulse
~ Moistens the lungs, stops phlegm, and resolves cough
~ Clears heat and toxic fire
~ Alleviates pain and stops spasms
~ Harmonizes other herbs and is an antidote for poisoning

Honey-frying roots
Never more an alchemist
than over that wok

Turning metal into gold
Adding the "shi" to Gan Cao

Golden aroma
Every 2nd Saturday
Badge of my office

Huang Jing

King Solomon Seal Rhizome

黄精 (Osei)

Rhizoma Polygonati

Sweet, Neutral
LU, SP

~ Tonifies the spleen Qi and stomach Yin
~ Moistens the lungs and generates lung Yin
~ Tonifies the kidneys, strengthen Jing, and relieves wasting

---

Solomon's keyring;
Doodles in the Bible margins
A bundle of roots

What Devil could not be tamed
By a man who loves plants and art

His source of power?
That he loved the creator
more than creation

Huang Qi

Astragalus, Milk-Vetch Root
黄耆 (Ogi)
Radix Astragali

Sweet, Slightly Warm
LU, SP

~ Tonifies spleen Qi and blood
~ Strengthens the spleen, and raises Yang Qi of spleen and stomach
~ Tonifies the Wei Qi, stabilizes the exterior, and tonifies the lungs
~ Tonifies Qi and blood due to loss of blood
~ Promotes discharge of pus, expels urine, drains edema, and
  generates flesh

For a chill in the spring
Huang Qi over Ren Shen
Heat over fire

Don't stoke the fireplace
a blanket will do

When cold to the bone
warm yourself by the fire
but don't linger there

Ren Shen

Ginseng Root

人参 (ninjin)

Radix Panax Ginseng

Sweet, Slightly Bitter, Slightly Warm
LU, SP

~ Very, strongly tonifies Yuan Qi,
~ Tonifies spleen, stomach, and lung Qi
~ Generates fluids and stops thirst
~ Tonifies the heart Qi and calms the spirit

Never-ending
Gnidne-reven
Reincarnation

Endless dentist appointment
Endless reasons to smile

Living forever
Does not sounds nearly as fun as
Living forever

Shan Yao

Mountain Yam Rhizome
山薬 (Sanyak)
Rhizoma Dioscoreae

Sweet, Neutral
KI, LU, SP

~ Tonifies the spleen and stomach Yin
~ Tonifies the lung Qi and Yin
~ Strengthens the kidney Yin and Jing

Sweet potato fries
Will you be a remedy
in 2,000 years?

Innovation to folk cure
Folk cure to innovation

"Science found it works!"
Was it really discovered,
or rediscovered

Tai Zi Shen

Prince Ginseng, Pseudostellaria Root
Radix Pseudostellariae

Sweet, Slightly Bitter, Neurtal
LU, SP

~   Strengthen the spleen and tonifies Qi
~   Tonifies lung Qi and stops spontaneous sweating
~   Generates fluids

The tiny ruler
drooling over his scepter
playing with his foot

How could someone so helpless
be so helpful to my heart

Looking at scrapbooks
Remembering royalty
is always royal

Herbs That Tonify Yang

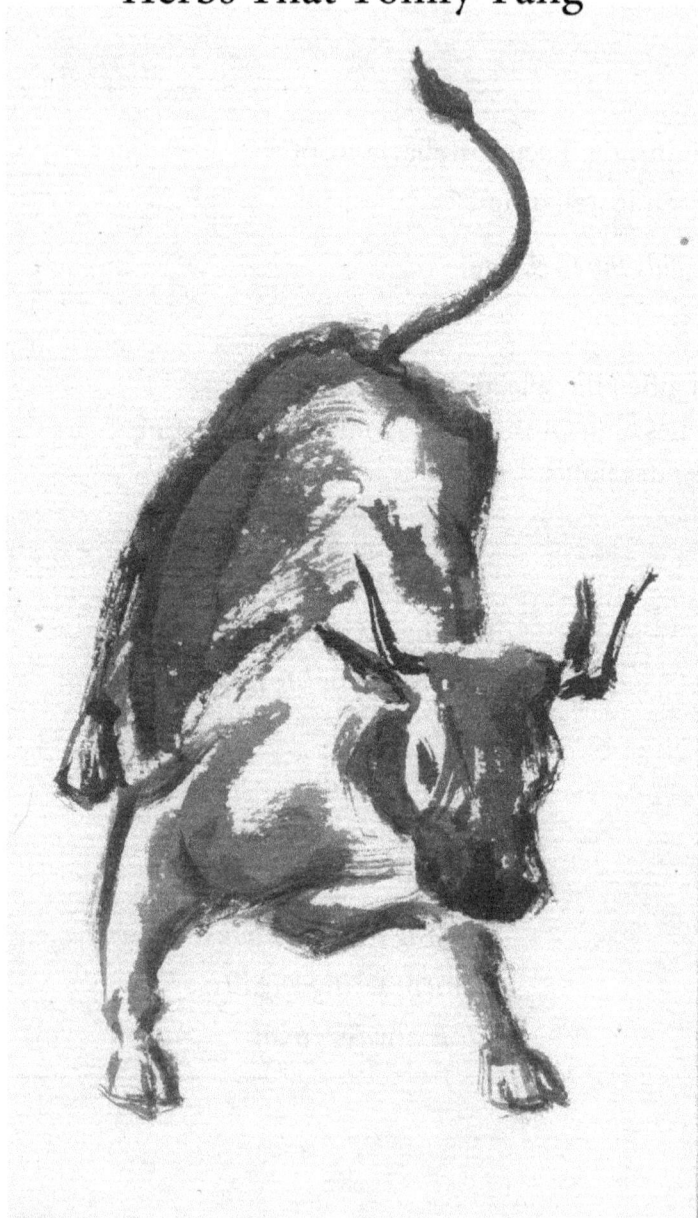

Ba Ji Tian

Morinda Root
Radix Morindae Officinalis

Spicy, Sweet, Slightly Warm
KI

~ Tonifies kidneys, reinforces sinews and bones and strengthens Yang
~ Expel wind damp cold

Scrubbing out a gash
with an old potato brush
into a mop sink

An aluminum kettle
over kerosene burner

Blue-tinted snapshots.
This is how I remember
the old man at work

Bu Gu Zhi

Scurf Pea, Psoraliae Fruit
Fructus Psoraliae

Bitter, Spicy, Hot
KI, SP

~ Tonifies the kidneys, strengthens Yang, and stabilizes Jing
~ Tonifies and strengthen spleen yang and stops diarrhea
~ Aids the kidneys to grasp lung Qi

On the field by 12
In the tractor by 14
Awake by 7

Quiet kids from the country
Cannot till the 405

In a 9 to 5
Their bank account grows zeros
That are worth nothing

Dong Chong Xia Cao

Chinese Caterpillar Fungus
冬虫夏草 (Tochukaso)
Cordyceps

Sweet, Warm
LU, KI

~ Strengthens the kidneys, fortifies Jing, and tonifies Yang
~ Nourish lung Yin, transform phlegm, stop cough, and arrests bleeding
~ Tonifies Yin and Yang

Quick growth and then death
Executives and fungus
have this in common

Both of them steering their host
from the dark into the red

There is no malice
Only the biology
of greed

Du Zhong

Eucommia Bark

杜仲 (Tochu)

Cortex Eucommiae

Sweet, Slightly Spicy, Warm
KI, LIV

~ Tonifies the liver and kidneys and strengthen sinews and bones
~ Promotes smooth flow of qi and blood and lowers blood pressure
~ Tonifies kidney Yang and eases dizziness

Beneath the armor
defenses for the vain eyes
A layer of silk

Bravery has its limits
in the socialites eyes

Brocades and chain mail
Suiting up for battle
On my way to school

Ge Jie

Toad-Headed Lizard

蛤蚧 (Gokai)

Gecko

Salty, Neutral, Slightly Toxic
LU, KI

~ Strengthen kidneys, tonifies lungs, and relieves cough
~ Tonifies Jing and blood, controls and stabilizes kidney Qi, and
  stabilizes Ming Men fire

Sits perfectly still
Perfecting Buddha Nature
For 12 million years

Yet when death or hunger loom
the lower brain takes over

Mara's flys buzzing
A pink bolt of lightning
Satori supper

Gou Ji

Chain Fern, Scythian Lamb Rhizome
Rhizoma Cibotii

Bitter, Sweet, Warm
KI, LIV

~ Tonifies liver and kidneys and strengthens sinews and bones
~ Expels wind, damp, and cold
~ Warms and stabilizes the Kidneys and prevents leakage

Lamb is a "warm" food
But does that come from its meat
Or from its nature

Its nature is to give heat
From its wool, flesh, and spirit

I sometimes feel guilt
for taking such offerings
that can't be returned

Gu Sui Bu

Boneknit Root
Rhizoma Drynariae

Bitter, Warm
KI, LIV

~ Tonifies kidney Yang, strengthens the sinews and bones, and
  benefits the ears
~ Mends injury to sinews and bones
~ Stimulates growth of hair and activates the blood

Twix prairie and sky
the cowboy's two medicines
Boneknit and whiskey

A cast made of resistance
and a boot made of leather

The boss is looking
at a resume of scars
written on his flesh

Hu Tao Ren

Walnut
Semen Juglandis

Sweet, Warm
KI, LI, LU

~ Tonifies Kidneys, restores the Jing, and strengthens weak back and knees
~ Astringes and warms the lungs, resolves cold phlegm, helps the kidney grasp lung Qi, and stops chronic cough and wheezing
~ Moisten intestines and unblocks the bowels

"Barbarian nut"
Swinging hammers through the walls
Surging in and out

The stale flavor of peace
Fat and pale like a peach Pit

We welcome defeat;
The hoard, bringing hot chaos
The hoard, bringing life

Lu Jiao Jiao

Deer Antler Glue
Gelatinum Cornu Cervi

Salty, Sweet, Warm
KID, LIV

~ Tonifies kidney Yang and Jing
~ Stops bleeding and treats Yin sores

The armor of war
Bloody rust gone, shining clean
At the mall's knife shop

Plastic curiosity
For cubical warriors

No one will buy it
But everyone will touch it
Shop owner chagrin

Lu Rong

Dear Antler Velvet
鹿茸 (Rokujo)
Cornu Cervi Pantotrichum

Salty, Sweet, Warm
KI, LIV

~ Tonifies kidneys and strengthen Yang
~ Tonifies the governing vessel, augments Jing and blood, and strengthens sinews and bones
~ Regulates the conception vessel and stabilizes the Dai Mai
~ Tonifies and nourishes Qi and blood and heals Yin type sores

---

Wearing dad's sweater
I'm amazed how it fits me
and how warm it is

I see him in the first row
Eyes on me, grey stripes on black

At the discount store
I see a stack of fathers
with an acrylic smell

Rou Cong Rong

Desert-Living Cistanche
(Nikujuyo) 肉苁容
Herba Cistanches

Salty, Sweet, Warm
KI, LI

~ Tonifies kidneys, strengthen yang, and improves the condition of
  marrow and Jing
~ Moistens the intestines and helps pass stool

Standing and blooming
with mindless vitality
Don Juan in the sand

"You must toss away logic"
and the logic of logic"

Reason is the lie
that steals magic from flowers
and poison from death

Sha Yuan Zi

Astragalus Seed – flattened
Semen Astragali Complanati

Sweet, Warm
KI, LI

~ Tonifies kidney yang, strengthen liver blood, and secures failing Jing

---

Even exhausted
Restless bouncing energy
springs from my godson

Chasing phantoms with flashlights
and booboos with bandages

The hot and glowing
will decay and stabilize
against my wishes

Suo Yang

Lock-*Yang* Stem

Herba Cynomorii

Sweet, Warm
KI, LI, LIV

~ Tonifies kidney Yang
~ Nourish blood, tonifies Jing and liver Yin, and strengthen sinews and marrow
~ Moisten intestines and opens the bowel

Every Saturday
I reaffirm my manhood
with beer and pretzels

Our chalice; the firepit
and our hymnal; an iPhone

Though the truth be told
I don't like the taste of beer
or pretzel gluten

Tu Si Zi

Chinese Dodder Seeds
Semen Cuscutae

Spicy, Sweet, Neutral
KI, LIV

~ Tonifies the kidneys and liver, strengthens Yin and Yang, secures
  Jing, and reserves urine
~ Strengthen the spleen and resolve diarrhea.
~ Calms the fetus in cases of habitual or threatened miscarriage.

On a green spring day
the pharmacy turned black
with tactical vests

They left us the Ephedra
and the marijuana seeds

Yet tiny dodder
was their primary target.
Cannon for mosquito

Xian Mao

Curculigo , Golden Eye-Grass Rhizome
Rhizoma Curculiginis

Spicy, Hot, Toxic
KI, LIV

~ Tonifies the kidneys and strengthens Yang
~ Expels cold and eliminates damp from sinews and bones

Xian Mao makes a trade;
For a longer life-maker
he'll shorten your life.

Growing in the Blackwater
Expelling cold, at a price

Sometimes old men think
It is better to burn up
than to fade away

Xu Duan

Himalayan Teasel Root
Radix Dipsaci

Bitter, Spicy, Sweet, Slightly Warm
KI, LIV

~ Tonifies liver and kidney and strengthen sinews and bones
~ Stops uterine bleeding and calms the fetus
~ Promotes blood circulation, alleviates pain, and generates flesh

---

She always paid me.
Even with an empty purse
and maxed out credit

A teacher with no students
still opens the school each day

One hopes for plenty
Though one can aspire to
g e n e r o s i t y

Yi Zhi Ren

Black Cardamon, Alpinia Fruit
Fructus Alpiniae Oxyphyllae

Spicy, Warm
KI, SP

~ Warms the kidneys, retains the Jing, and holds urine
~ Warms the spleen, stops diarrhea, and stimulates the appetite

---

Indian buffet
Even after a whole year
they don't trust my taste

Their lunch, pungent and simple
My lunch, a show for tourists

The bearded owner
Without a word brings me chai
I'm in, but not in

Yin Yang Huo

Horny Goat Weed Leaf
淫羊藿 (Inyokaku)
Herba Epimedii

Spicy, Sweet, Warm
KI, LIV

~ Tonifies the kidneys and Yang
~ Expel wind damp, cold
~ Strengthen Yin and Yang, anchors down liver Yang rising

Leaves bound like money
and worth every penny
Epimedii leaf

Grandpa Simpson's tonic secret:
Bourbon and Horny Goat Weed

Sometimes compassion
comes in a brown paper bag
filled with stems and leaves

Herbs That Tonifies Yin

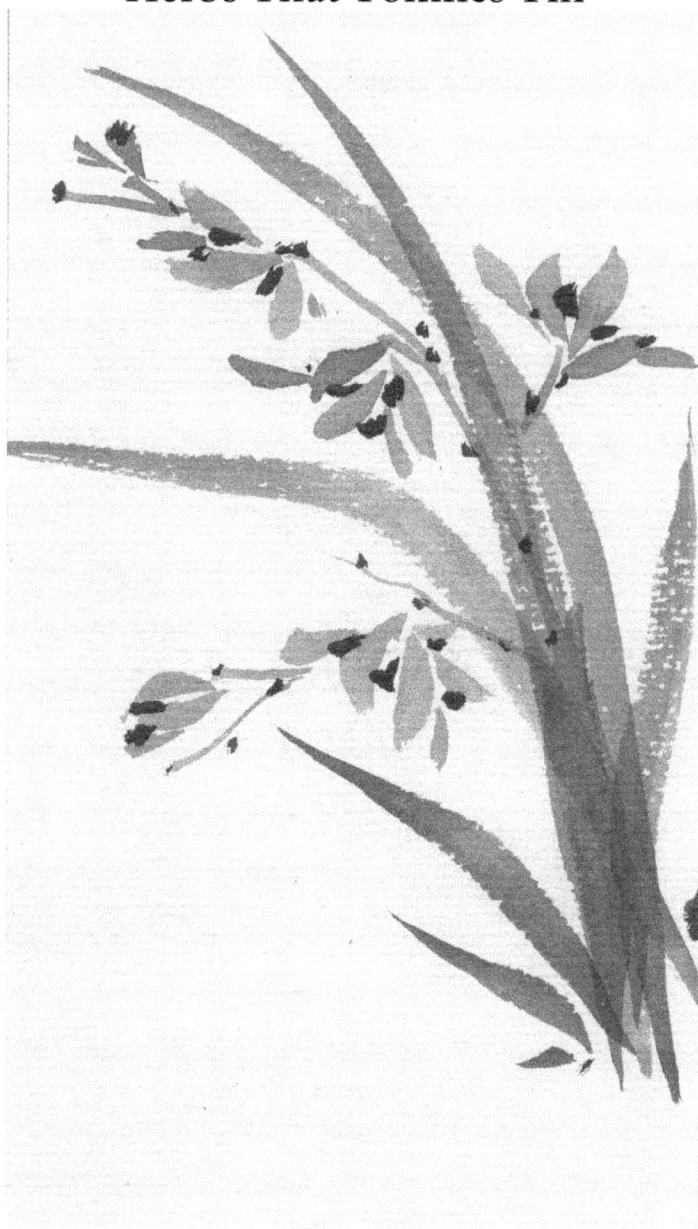

Bai He

Tiger Lily Bulb
百合 (Byakugo)
Bulbus Lilii

Sweet, Slightly Bitter, Cool
HRT, LU

~ Moistens the lungs, nourishes Yin, clears heat, and stops coughing
~ Calms the spirit, nourishes stomach Yin, and harmonizes the middle Jiao

---

Only one takes root
from the garden waste gully
The Tiger Lilly

A mouth full of stamens
A roar full of pollen

Driven to the sun
Clawing up the embankment
one bloom at a time

Bie Jia

Chinese Soft-Shell Turtle Shell
Carapax Amydae / Trionycis

Salty, Slightly Cold
LIV, SP

~ Nourish Yin and anchor Yang
~ Invigorates the blood, promotes menses, and dissipates nodules
~ Heavily anchors, assists, and unblocks the blood vessels

From our honeymoon
I remember tortoises
and pizza on cardboard

Seaweed that looked like serpents
Tiger cowries and kava

Rickety kayak
Busses on bridges for bikes
Endless brittle stars

Gui Ban

Freshwater Turtle Shell
Plastrum Testudinis

Salty, Sweet, Cold
HRT, KI, LIV

~ Nourishes Yin and anchor yang
~ Resolves liver and kidney Yin deficiency
~ Benefits the kidneys and strengthens bones
~ Cools the blood and stops uterine bleeding due to heat
~ Tonifies the blood, nourishes and calms the heart

In Geode Canyon
What I thought was a viper
was a turtle shell

Snapping at my plastic bait
Papi snapping back at me

Left in the front yard
Picked up by a neighbor dog
and carried away

Han Lian Cao

Field Lotus Herb
Herba Ecliptae

Sour, Sweet, Slightly Cold
KI, LIV

~ Enriches the liver and kidney Yin
~ Cools blood and stops bleeding

What grows in the field
And what grows in the mire
Bloom with soft sweetness

Both strive to please each other
with no concept of a mirror

But to scientists
there's no dichotomy key
for love and beauty

Hei Zhi Ma

Black Sesame Seed
Semen Sesame Indici

Sweet, Neutral
KI, LI, LIV

~ Tonifies the Yin of the liver and kidney systems
~ Nourish liver blood and Jing
~ Moisten and lubricate the intestines

Desperate for a snack
I mix sesame and salt
with red vinegar

When my student loans are due
Condiments become courses

My degree left unfinished
Like salt, vinegar,
and black sesames

358

Luo Han Guo

Momordica Fruit

Fructus Momordicae

Sweet, Neutral
LI, LU

~ Moistens and cools the lungs, clears phlegm, dissipates nodules, and soothes cough
~ Generates fluids, moistens the intestines, relieves thirst, and unblocks the bowels

---

Rediscovery!
Something we've known for years
Seen in a new light

What benefitted the throat
Now benefits the pallet

The green light of cash
makes a lot of remedies
into medicine

Mai Men Dong

Ophiopogon tuber
麦門冬 (Bakumondo)
Radix Ophiopogonis

Sweet, Slightly Bitter, Slightly Cold
HRT, LU, ST

~ Moistens the lungs, nourishes Yin, and stops cough
~ Augments stomach Yin and generates fluids
~ Clears heat and eliminates irritability due to Yin deficiency
~ Moistens the intestines

A crying baby
Makes me forget my problems:
Homeopathy

In the Universe's eye
we are equally helpless

Crying with infants
They convey their sympathies
without any words

Nu Zhen Zi

Privet Fruit
Fructus Ligustri Lucidi

Bitter, Sweet, Cool
KI, LIV

~ Enriches kidney and liver Yin
~ Clears deficient heat and improves vision

My heart kept hidden
Behind the leaf barrier
Green preventing green

Plumes of white flowers
Showy for showiness sake

All my false efforts
in saponin berries
fit for birds and fools

Sang Ji Sheng

Mistletoe stems
Herba Taxilli

Bitter, Sweet, Neutral
KI, LIV

~ Tonifies liver and kidney Yin, strengthen sinews and bones, and
  expels wind damp
~ Nourish blood, benefits the skin, and calms the womb

My dear frozen friend
How much wormwood you will need
to thaw out your heart

Embers in artimesia
false smoke and giraffe mailbox

Ignoring the bridge
where carp and children swim
we forded the Platte

Bei Sha Shen

Four Leaf Lady-Bell Root
浜防風 (hamabofu)
Radix Glehniae

Sweet, Slightly Bitter, Slightly Cold
LU, ST

~ Moistens the lungs, enriches lung Yin, and stops cough
~ Nourish the stomach Yin and generate fluids
~ Tonifies liver and kidney Yin
~ Moisten the skin and exterior

On my dresser mirror
notes taken from a movie
On how to fall in love

Longing looks and a slow waltz
A kiss that makes me real

Not a week later
the folded note went missing.
Taking notes on shame

Shi Hu

Stonebushel Stem
石斛 (Sekkoku)
Herba Dendrobii

Sweet, Slightly Salty, Bland, Slightly Cold
KI, ST

~ Nourishes Yin, clears heat, and generates fluids
~ Clears deficient heat and nourishes Yin in the lower jiao
~ Tonifies the kidneys, augments Jing, and brightens the eyes
~ Strengthens the tendons and bones and strengthens the low back

---

For extending life
There are few remedies
good as gardening

Replacing weeks with flowers
Trading stones for their essence

Back turned to the sun
axes flying, blades plunging
war with the barbarous Earth

Tian Men Dong

Shiny Asparagus Tuber
Radix Asparagi

Bitter, Sweet, Very Cold
KI, LU

~ Nourishes kidney Yin, sedates fire, and clears lung heat
~ Moistens the lungs, nourishes the kidneys, generates fluids, and
  resolves phlegm

Buried treasure found!
Asparagus and morels
underneath the pine

How come the grocery market
is trusted more than the soil?

The fear of poison
overcomes my thriftiness
and my hunger pangs

Xi Yang Shen

American Ginseng Root
Radix Panax Quinquefolii

Sweet, Slightly Bitter, Cold
HRT, KI, LU

~ Enriches Qi, generates fluids, and nourishes Yin
~ Nurtures lung Yin and clears fire from the lungs
~ Sedates heat in the intestines and stops bleeding

Teenage heritage;
Yellow soda and french fries
Eaten in green rooms

Clove cigarettes and mocha
The smell of my first car

These things, now plastic.
Brominated oil, trans fats
Cancer, caffeine, crusher

Yu Zhu

Fragrant Solomon's Seal Root
Rhizoma Polygonati Odorati

Sweet, Slightly Cold
LU, ST

~ Nourish Yin, moisten lung dryness, generates fluids, and
  nourishes the stomach
~ Stops wind and softens and moistens the sinews

The merchant witches
selling pewter pentagrams
on nylon cordage

Geomancy and taxes
wax idols made in China

When equally loved
Unicorn horn and plastic
share the same power

Herbs That Transform Phlegm Cold

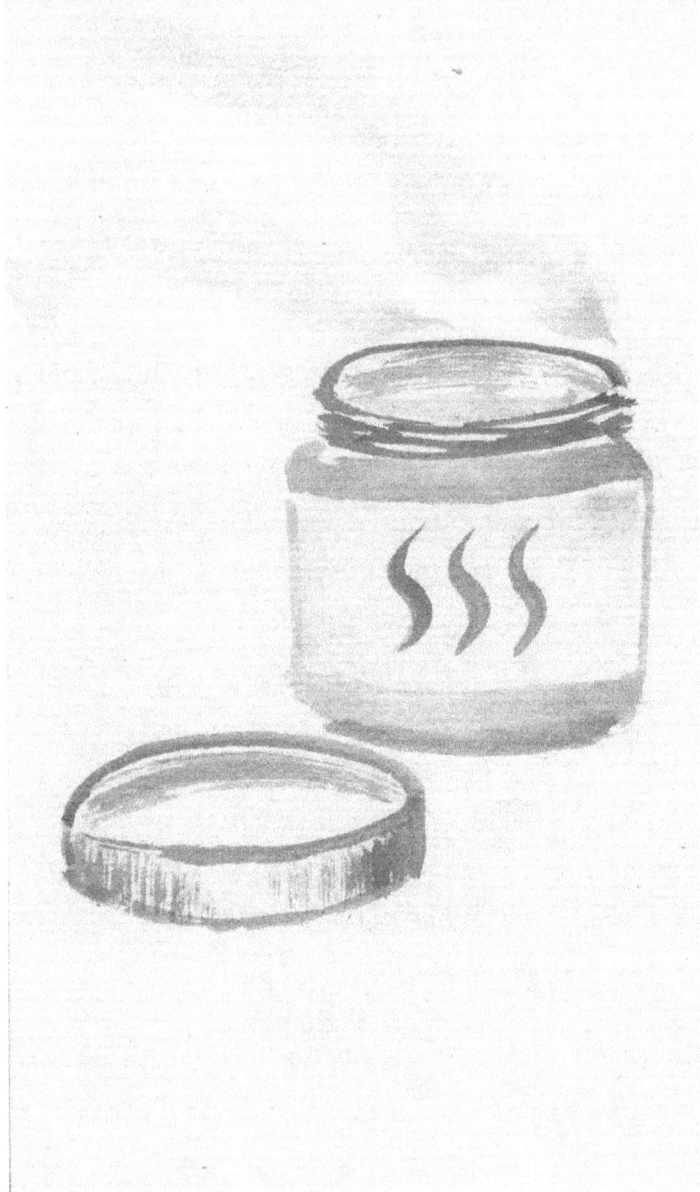

Bai Fu Zi

Giant Typhonium Rhizome
Rhizoma Typhonii Preparatum

Spicy, Sweet, Warm, Toxic
LIV, SP, ST

~ Dries dampness, transforms phlegm, expels wind, and stops spasms
~ Relieves toxicity and dissipates nodules
~ Dries dampness and stops pain

I wish for a flood
to wash away the garbage
on the banks of my heart

Love notes and plastic bottles
damming my tributaries

Open up your gates
and wash me away
until there is just us

Bai Jie Zi

White Mustard Seed
Semen Sinapis

Spicy, Warm
LU

~ Warms the lungs, regulates Qi, and expels phlegm
~ Moves Qi, dissipates nodules, reduces swelling, alleviates pain, and unblocks the collaterals

---

"Perfect white mustard"
Ingredient or puja?
I don't remember

Grey Poupon on my hot dog
a sacrament to summer

A secret passage
across the neglected park
7-11

Bai Qian

Willow Leaf Swallow Wort Rhizome
Rhizoma Cynanchi Stauntonii

Spicy, Sweet, Slightly Warm
LU

~   Redirects lung Qi downward, expels phlegm, and stops cough

---

Under the Platte's bridge
Potters have been hard at work
Daubing mud on rails

Successive generations
A history of pinch pots

Out pops a bird head
An artist in residence
belting a new tune

Ban Xia

Pinellia corm
半夏 (Hange)
Rhizoma Pinelliae Preparatum

Spicy, Warm, Toxic
LU, SP, ST

~ Dries dampness and transforms cold phlegm
~ Anchors rebellious stomach QI and stops vomiting
~ Dissipates nodules and reduces distension and stagnation
~ Treats hot sores on the surface

An angry child
instantly pacified
by Grandma's cookie

Her legacy is written
in a box of index cards

There's no grave cleaning
Just the hand-rolling of dough
and pounds of butter

Jie Geng

Balloon Flower Root
桔梗 (Kikyo)
Radix Platycodi

Biter, Spicy, Neutral
LU

~ Opens up and spreads lung Qi, expels phlegm, benefits the throat and voice
~ Promotes discharge of pus
~ Guides other herbs to the upper body

Karaoke man:
Bohemian Rhapsody
lures me to join in

Intoxicated by song
Embarrassment hangover

Only the truly mad
those few, with stars in their eyes
can take to the stage

Tian Nan Xing

Jack-in-the-Pulpit, Dragon Arum corm

天南星 (Tennansho)

Rhizoma Arisaematis Preparatum

Bitter, Spicy, Warm Toxic
LIV, LU, SP

~ Dries dampness and expels phlegm
~ Disperses wind phlegm in the channels and stops spasms
~ Reduces swelling and alleviates pain topically

A tiny dragon
hidden in the petal folds
roaring with beauty

Across the deep Pacific
Phantoms turn into preachers

A floral preacher
upon creation's pulpit
spitting hot fire

Xuan Fu Hua

Japanese Elecampane Flower

旋覆花 (Senpukuka)

Flos Inulae

Bitter, Salty, Spicy, Slightly Warm
LIV, LU, SP, ST

~ Resolves phlegm stagnation in the lungs and dries pathogenic waters
~ Stops rebellious Qi in the stomach

Traveling elf-herb
from the emerald Isles
to the giant's teat

The icy tears of Helen
Heal both horses and humans

Fragrant legacy
from the dinner of Pliny
to the chemist's desk

Zao Jiao

Chinese Honeylocust Fruit
Fructus Gleditsiae

Spicy, Warm, Slightly Toxic
LU, LI

~ Dispels phlegm and phlegm nodules
~ Opens the orifices and revives the spirit
~ Dissipates clumps and reduces swellings.

Is tomorrow's health
worth an injury today?
Spiny Gleditsia

Both Adonis and glutton
fall before a Cadillac

There is no gamble
if living in the present
in comfortable flesh

Zao Jiao Ci

Chinese Honey Locust thorn
Spina Gleditsiae

Spicy, Warm
LIV, LU, ST

~ Draws out toxicity, discharges pus, invigorates blood, reduces
  abscesses and swelling
~ Expels wind and kills parasites

Her scalpel fingers
occasionally augmented
by a dull wood thorn

Kneading knots back into rope
and scars back into muscle

Blunted instruments
and an unfocused doctor
at the mall's masseuse

Herbs That Warm the Interior and Expel Cold

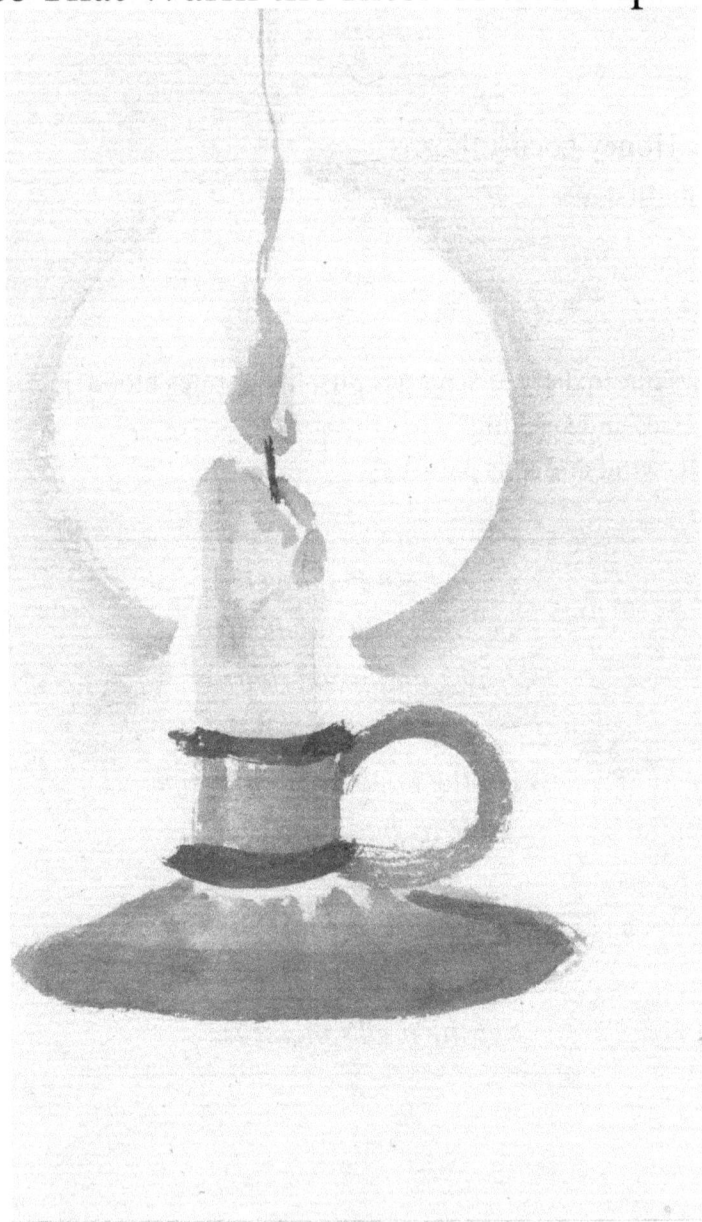

Chuan Jiao

Chinese Prickly-Ash, Sichuan Peppercorn
Pericarpium Zanthoxyli

Spicy, Hot, Slightly Toxic
KI, SP, ST

~ Warms the middle Jiao, disperses cold, dries dampness, and calms
  vomiting and diarrhea
~ Kills parasites and relieves abdominal pain

Laughing and burning
We prepare Sichuan cuisine
over his divorce

All the Asian peppercorns
numb the spice but not the pain

Looking to the day
where we have so much joy
we can piss it away

Ding Xiang

Clove

丁香 (Choko)

Flos Caryophylli

Spicy, Warm

KI, SP, ST

~ Warms the middle burner, directs rebellious Qi downward, and
  alleviates pain
~ Warms the kidneys and boost Yang

A worm in my tooth
I stop it from turning
Chewing on clavos

The taste of fresh pumpkin pie
masked by a numbed tongue

Woody flower bulb
From the sultans to the dentists
a gift to mankind

Fu Zi

Sichuan Aconite Root
附子 (Bu Shi)
Radix Aconiti Lateralis

Spicy, Very Hot, Toxic
HRT, KI, SP

~ Restores devastated Yang and rescues it from rebellion
~ Assists heart Yang to unblock vessels, tonifies kidney and spleen
  Yang to augment fire
~ Warms fire and assists Yang
~ Disperses cold, warms the channels, and alleviates pain

Blind with schoolyard rage
I lash out against the world
and tackle my bully

My knuckles cut on his teeth
Pollock painting in blood and tears

Mid-punch, white then black
Heart pounding disappointment
Alarm clock buzzing

Gan Jiang

Dried Ginger Rhizome
乾姜 (Kankyo)
Rhizoma Zingiberis

Spicy, Hot
HRT, LU, SP, ST

~ Warms the middle, insulates the lower Jiao, and expels cold
~ Rescues devastated Yang and expels interior cold
~ Warms the lungs and transforms thin phlegm
~ Warms the channels, stops bleeding, and unblocks the pulse

On the windowsill
behind the desktop tower
A stalk of ginger

In a jar of stale water
a slice of root from Kroger's

Trapped in the 'burbs
An exotic mystery
growing on nothing

Gao Liang Jiang

Lesser Galangal Rhizome
Rhizoma Alpiniae Officinarum

Spicy, Hot
SP, ST

~ Warms the middle Jiao, alleviates pain, and disperses congestive
   Qi

I cannot resist
a cook who calls me "my friend"
and offers me food

If he says the lamb kebab
I'm on vegan suspension

He asks if it is good
knowing the only answer
"yes, it's delicious"

Rou Gui

Cassia Cinnamon Bark
Cortex Cinnamomi

Spicy, Sweet, Hot
HRT, KI, LIV, SP

~ Warms the kidneys, spleen, and heart, strengthens Yang and Ming Men fire
~ Leads floating yang back to its source
~ Disperses deep cold, warms and unblocks the channels, and alleviates pain
~ Leads the fire back to its source and encourages generation of Qi and blood

---

Adventure for kids
Nostalgia for parents
Cinnamon flavor

How did a tropical Bark
come to taste like Christmas?

How did the King's Spice
go from being paid in blood
to candied for nickels

Wu Zhu Yu

Evodia Fruit
吳茱萸 (Goshuyu)
Fructus Evodiae

Bitter, Spicy, Hot, Slightly Toxic
LIV, SP, ST

~ Warms the middle Jiao, disperses cold, relieves constrained Qi movement, and relieves pain
~ Redirects stomach Qi downwards and stops vomiting
~ Warms the spleen, expels damp cold, and stops diarrhea.
~ Leads fire downwards from the mouth and tongue

Lacking Goshuyu,
Pull up the skin on the spine
In rows like ladder rungs

A lesson from Abuela
A secret that I'm sharing

Hidden recipes
and Die Da Jiao formulas
Toss them in the light

Xiao Hui Xiang

Fennel Fruit

茴香 (Uikyo)

Fructus Foeniculi

Spicy, Warm
KI, LIV, SP, ST

~   Spreads liver Qi, warms the kidneys and liver, and alleviates pain
~   Regulates Qi and harmonizes the stomach

A dose of fennel
in my toothpaste and desserts
assures ownership

The only one in my troup
who takes bitter with cloying

Never matching tastes
with my home society
or the ones I love

Index

www.ingramcontent.com/pod-product-compliance
Lightning Source LLC
Chambersburg PA
CBHW031457270326
41930CB00006B/136